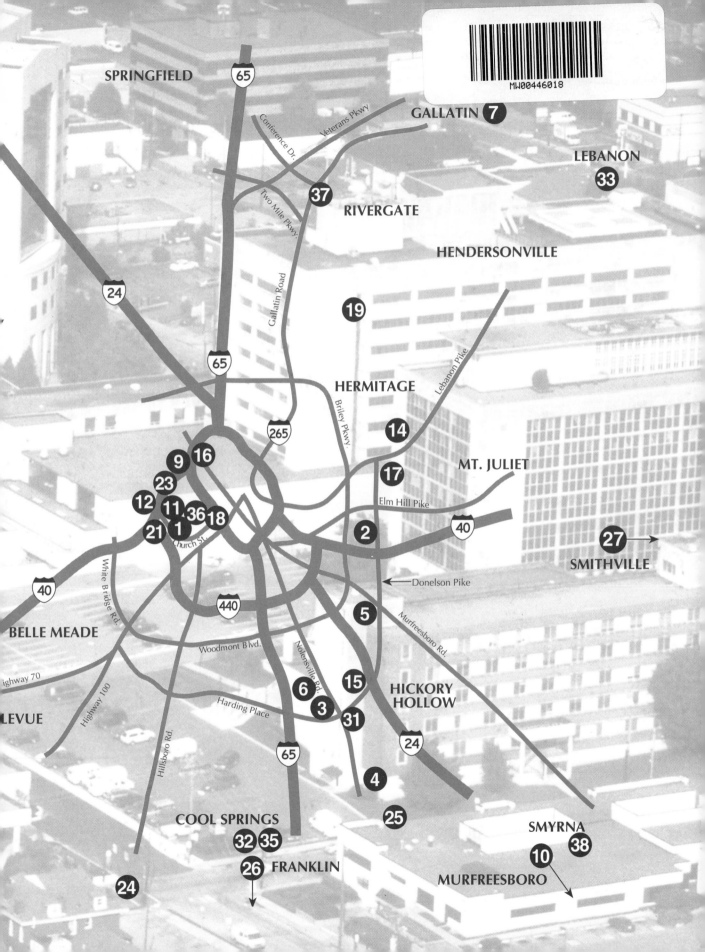

SPRINGFIELD

65

GALLATIN **7**

Conference Dr.

Veterans Pkwy.

24

Two Mile Pkwy.

37

RIVERGATE

LEBANON

33

HENDERSONVILLE

Gallatin Road

19

65

HERMITAGE

Lebanon Pike

265

Briley Pkwy.

14

9 **16**

17

MT. JULIET

23

12

11 **36** **18**

Elm Hill Pike

21 **1**

Church St.

2

40

27

SMITHVILLE

Donelson Pike ←

White Bridge Rd.

40

BELLE MEADE

440

5

Murfreesboro Rd.

ighway 70

Woodmont Blvd.

LEVUE

Highway 100

Harding Place

Nolensville Rd.

15

HICKORY
HOLLOW

Hillsboro Rd.

6

3

31

65

24

4

25

COOL SPRINGS

SMYRNA

32 **35**

38

26

FRANKLIN

10

24

MURFREESBORO

A Heritage of
Healing

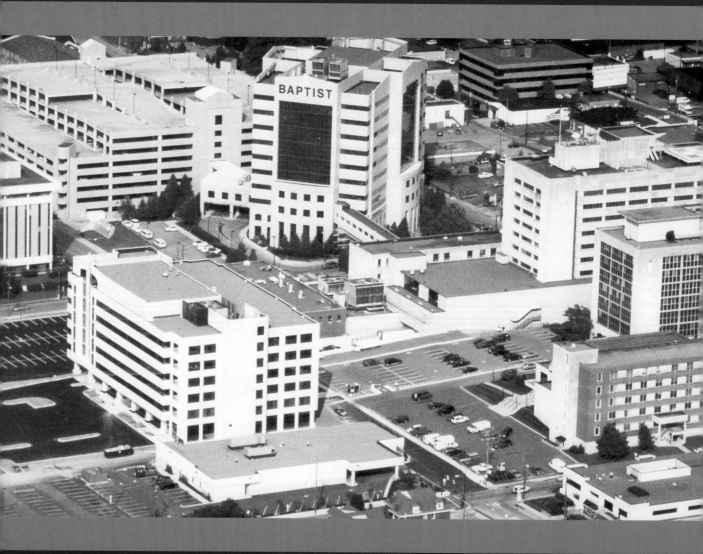

HILLSBORO PRESS

Franklin, Tennessee

A HERITAGE OF HEALING

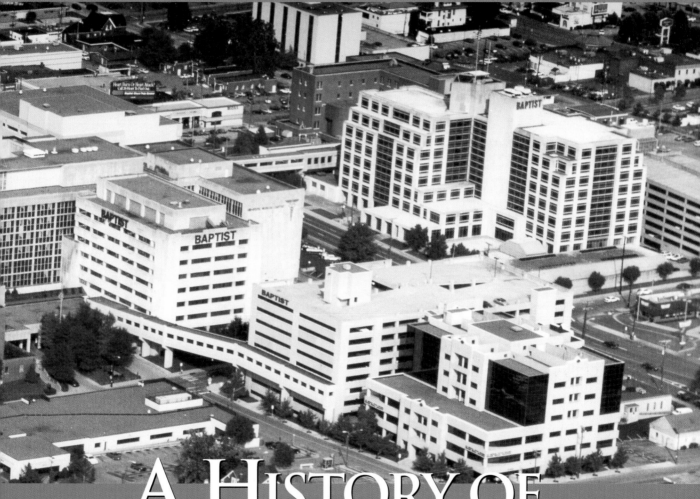

Serving Middle Tennessee at Many Locations

A HISTORY OF BAPTIST HOSPITAL

Nashville, Tennessee 1918-1998

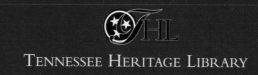

TENNESSEE HERITAGE LIBRARY

Library of Congress Catalog Card Number: 98-75321

ISBN: 1-57736-124-5

Bible version used is the New American Standard Bible.

Editorial Consultant: Dimples B. Kellogg
Cover design: Gary Bozeman

Photo Credits: Tennessee State Library and Archives, Massachusetts Commandery, Military Order of the Loyal Legion and the U.S. Army Military History Institute, Jack Gunter, Dana Thomas, Owen Cartwright, Earl Warren Jr., Bill Lokey

Published by
HILLSBORO PRESS
An imprint of
PROVIDENCE HOUSE PUBLISHERS
238 Seaboard Lane • Franklin, Tennessee 37067
800-321-5692

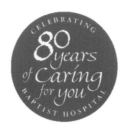

TO THE THOUSANDS OF MEN AND WOMEN who, over the past eighty years as part of this Christian healing ministry, have worked so hard and given so much to render to our patients and their families the highest quality of care in an exceptionally compassionate manner.

CONTENTS

PREFACE

BAPTIST HOSPITAL CELEBRATES ITS EIGHTIETH anniversary in 1998, and this book commemorates this milestone. In the course of those years, the hospital's name has changed from Protestant Hospital to Mid-State Baptist Hospital to Baptist Hospital. Its mission has remained the same, however. As a Christian healing ministry, Baptist Hospital is committed to rendering the highest quality health care in an exceptionally caring and compassionate atmosphere in the most efficient, cost-effective manner possible.

Many buildings and programs and technological advances are discussed in this historical look at the hospital. Yet individuals and their well-being are the reasons for their existence, and the people who have worked in the hospital or on its behalf have never overlooked this crucial point. Prominent among them has been David Stringfield, current president and CEO of Baptist Hospital, whose dedication and vision have guided the hospital to many notable accomplishments.

While serving in the position of chairman of the board, I have had the pleasure of working with the physicians, nursing staff and other employees, administration, and members of the board to meet the community's healthcare needs in recent years and prepare the hospital of the challenges of the next century. Perhaps the only certainty about health care in the coming years is that it will continue to change. Baptist hospital's position as the largest not-for-profit hospital in Middle Tennessee and its diversified programs and services make it ready to continue improving and enhancing the health of the community and doing work to the glory of God.

Guy E. Bates Sr.
Chairman, Board of Trustees
September 1998

Chapter One

EARLY DAYS

Nashville led the nation with its high death rate.
—Dr. John Berrien Lindsley
City health officer, 1877

THE AREA THAT WAS TO BECOME NASHVILLE, Tennessee, was occupied in 1200 with large Native American villages. By 1450 the villages had disappeared, and Native Americans used the area primarily for hunting.

Sometime in the 1600s Charleville, a French-Canadian fur trader, established a trading post at the French Lick. (The name of Nashville came into use when the town was officially established in 1784.) The post remained in place until 1714 when it was abandoned.

The Shawnee were the last tribe to try to settle the area, but the Chickasaw and Cherokee drove them out in 1715. More than fifty years later, in 1769, Timothy Demonbreun, a French-Canadian fur trader, began hunting at the French Lick.

When white pioneers arrived in 1779–80, Cherokee, Choctaw, Chickasaw, and Creek still used the area only for hunting, fishing, and trading. James Robertson led the first group of settlers, mostly men and boys. Colonel John Donelson with the women and children on flatboats were the next arrivals.

For many years the only doctors for the settlers were a horse doctor and Granny Nell, an older Shawnee woman who tended to women with "female problems" and ran a tavern on the square. Men swapped homemade prescriptions for ills such as rheumatism, fever, snake bite, tapeworm, and wounds from fights with Native Americans and one another. Smallpox hit the settlers in 1780, but there was little they could do.

An early community leader, not a physician, conducted the first operation. James Robertson performed "surgery" on David Hood after he had been scalped. In *Pioneer Medicine and Early Physicians*, Dr. T. V. Woodring described the procedure: Robertson took a "pegging awl and perforated thickly the whole naked space going through the outer table of the skull." Apparently he made the holes close together; then granulation covered the skull before the skull died. Hood lived for several years afterward.

Felix Robertson was the first white child born in what is now Metro Nashville. He was born at Freeland's Station (around 1400 Eighth Avenue North) on January 11, 1781. He became a physician and a professor of medicine at the University of Nashville. Robertson was the first native-born Nashvillian to graduate from medical college; the first physician in Nashville to specialize in pediatrics and to use quinine for malaria; the first mayor of Nashville elected by direct vote; and the first president of the city's board of health.

Some dispute seems to surround the issue of which physician was the first to arrive. Most sources identify Dr. John Sappington, and the date as 1785. A few state that Dr. James White preceded him in 1784 and that Sappington did not make his appearance until 1786. His brother Mark Sappington was also a doctor, as was Mark's son,

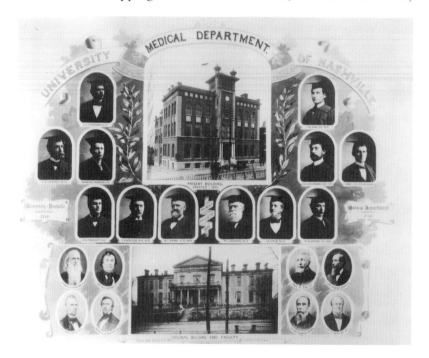

The Medical School of the University of Nashville was an early place of care for Nashvillians who were ill.

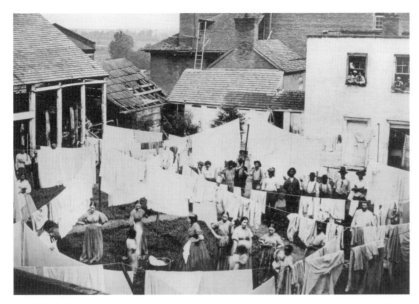

This hospital laundry yard in 1863 served only one of the many facilities in Nashville that was turned into a hospital during the Civil War.

Roger B. Sappington. Joining these physicians were Dr. John Shelby in 1785 (Shelby Medical College was named for him), Dr. Boyd McNairy in 1786, Dr. Francis May in 1790, and Dr. Charles K. Winston in 1811. Bleeding was the treatment of choice for most ills, even typhoid. A physician on his rounds had limited tools in his saddlebag, usually a knife or two, and he relied on assorted herbs for his pharmacy. Most physicians in Nashville sold medicine as well as practiced medicine.

Many people without qualifications or official training practiced medicine. Although efforts were made to enact a law to regulate the practice as early as 1817, licenses were not required to practice medicine in the state until 1889. In this regard Tennessee was not really behind the times; few states insisted on licensing physicians.

In 1821, physicians James Overton, Felix Robertson, John Waters, Boyd McNairy, R. A. Higginbotham, A. C. Goodlett, and James Roane standardized medical charges. Here are some examples: $1 for a visit in town; $1 for six pills; and $50 for an amputation. The group was a precursor of an organized medical society in Nashville.

People practiced medicine on themselves with the help of books written for laypersons. *Gunn's Domestic Medicine* was published from 1832 to 1838 in several editions, and *The Cherokee Physician or Indian Guide to Health, as given by Richard Foreman, a Cherokee-doctor* was published in 1846.

By 1850 the number of physicians had reached about three dozen. The community, which numbered 10,165 in the 1850 census,

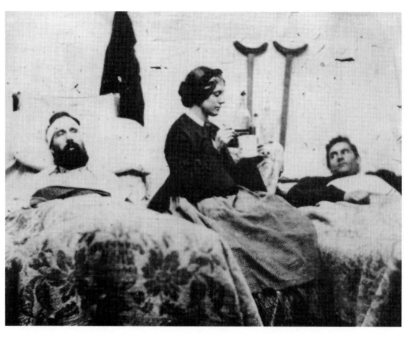

Nashville's hospitals were filled with wounded soldiers as a result of the war; here a Union nurse cares for patients.

probably could have used even more to battle cholera epidemics in 1850, 1854, and 1866. (There had also been one in 1849 and the one to come in 1873 would kill one thousand people.)

The decade of the 1850s saw other, more positive medical events. Central Hospital for the Insane was built in 1851 on the south side of Murfreesboro Pike. John Berrien Lindsley, A. H. Buchanan, Robert Porter, John M. Watson, W. K. Bowling, and Charles K. Winston organized Nashville Medical School; opening day was November 3, 1851. The American Medical Association held its national convention in Nashville in 1857 (and also in 1890).

The Civil War turned many Nashville institutions into hospitals; among them were hotels, such as Planter's Hotel at Fifth Avenue North and Deaderick, the Masonic Hall, and several churches. Twenty thousand women (mostly white but some slave women) performed nursing and support services at more than twenty Federal hospitals. The U.S. Sanitary Commission looked after both Federal and Confederate soldiers.

Dr. Winston was behind the formation of the first board of health in Nashville, established in 1866, but the board did not remain constant for many periods and public health suffered as a result of this deficiency. After the Civil War, several forces combined to adversely affect public health. So many newly freed black people poured into town that there was severe overcrowding in the North Nashville area. Other areas of town were equally overcrowded, particularly during the 1880s. By 1880, the population had grown to 43,350, and it would climb to 76,168 by 1890. Nashville had polluted wells, polluted air with lots of smoke, and poor to nonexistent sewerage disposal. Tuberculosis and pneumonia overcame people in slums because even damp basement rooms were rented out. Other too common killers were diphtheria, diarrhea, smallpox, measles, scarlet fever, typhoid, and malaria.

The founding of Meharry Medical College in 1876 was a boon to the community, especially in meeting the medical needs of the black population. In *Educating Black Doctors: A History of Meharry Medical College*, James Summerville noted that "its early students were former slaves or descendants of slaves." However, the city's General Hospital, with sixty beds, was not constructed until 1890. Before that the medical schools—University of Nashville, Nashville Medical School, Vanderbilt (its medical school opened in 1873 but it had no hospital until 1925), and Meharry—cared for people. One hundred years ago not-for-profit hospitals were completely charitable. Patients did not pay. Hospitals, many of them owned by churches, were for the destitute. Doctors made house calls to the wealthy.

Bishop Thomas Byrne of the Nashville Diocese bought the Jacob McGavock Dickinson estate between Hayes and Church Streets and present Twentieth and Twenty-first Avenues to build a Catholic

City Hospital of Nashville, later called General Hospital, was not built until 1890.

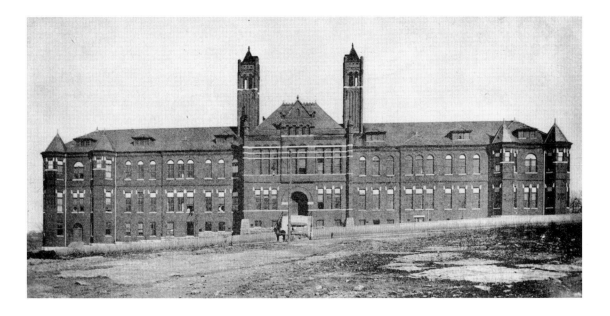

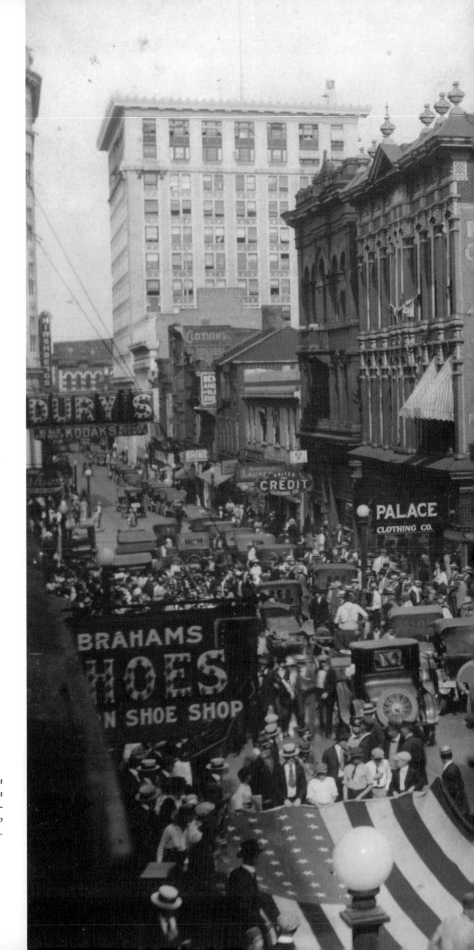

Nashvillians crowded into Union Street for a World War I rally in 1918. The city's growing population required more hospitals to meet medical needs.

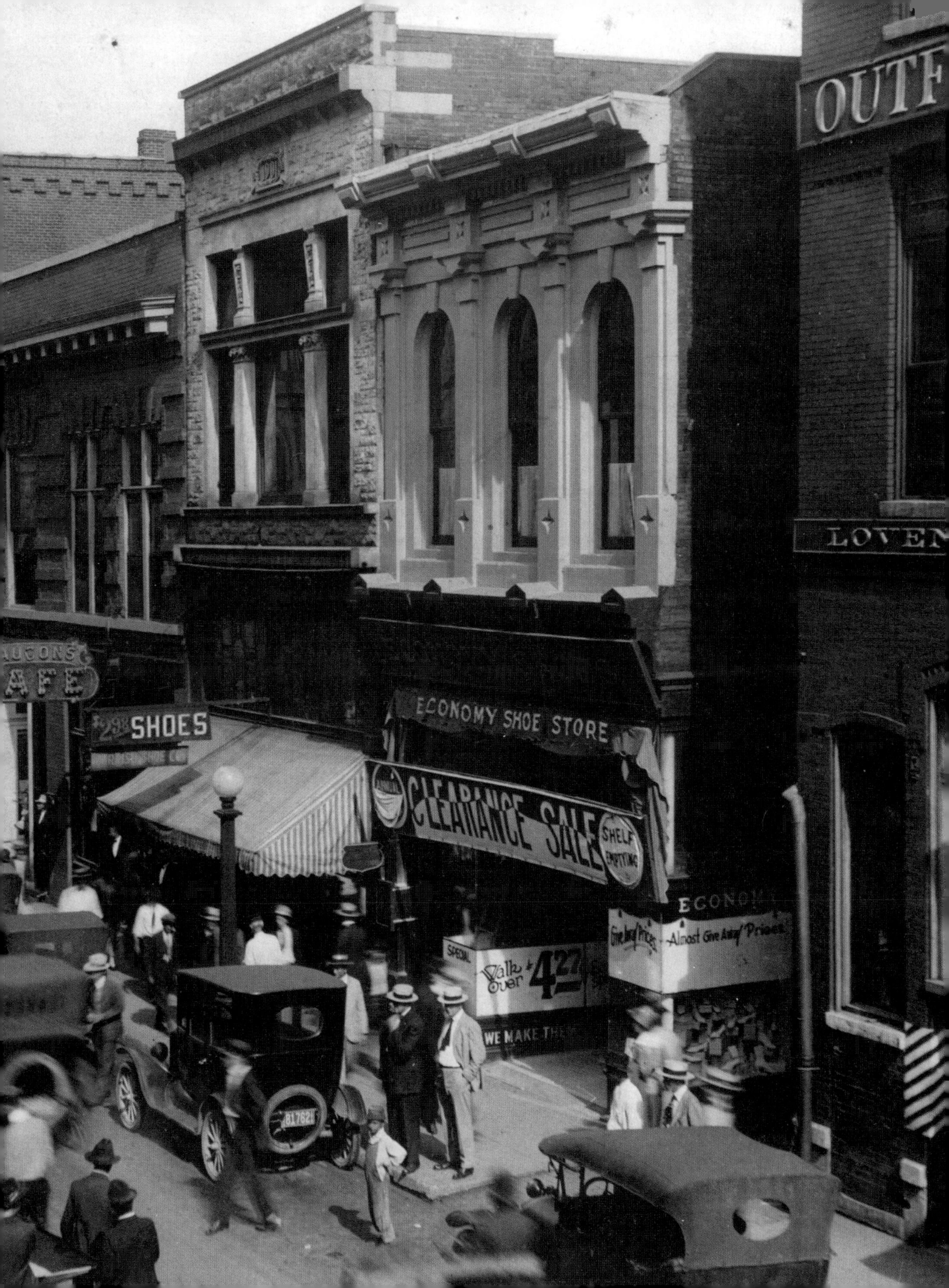
OUTF
LOVEN
SHOES
ECONOMY SHOE STORE
CLEARANCE SALE
SHELF EMPTYING
Almost Give Away Prices
SPECIAL
Walk Over 4.27
WE MAKE THE

hospital. In 1898 the Daughters of Charity of Saint Vincent DePaul opened Saint Thomas with twenty-six beds in the former Dickinson residence until a hospital could be built. The new five-story building received patients in 1902. The cost was $200,000, but its modern conveniences included telephones and electric elevators. Horse-drawn ambulances brought patients to the hospital.

In 1910 Meharry opened an unfinished George W. Hubbard Hospital. Meharry students were not allowed at Nashville General Hospital because of their race.

Polio was an ever-present fear in 1916. Nationwide there were 6,000 deaths and 27,000 people were paralyzed. Physicians could do little but comfort their patients.

Nashville's *1918 Classified Directory* lists the following health-related institutions: Briggs' Private Surgical Infirmary, 421 Third Avenue; City View Sanitarium, Murfreesboro Pike; Millie E. Hale Hospital (notes that it is colored), 523 Seventh Avenue; Highland Sanitarium, Route 7; Hite Home Sanitarium, 947–949 Russell Street; Nashville City Hospital, Nance Street; and Saint Thomas Hospital, 2000 Hayes Street.

The Nashville area, which had had a constant flow of new citizens, experienced a major influx of newcomers with the building of the town of Old Hickory and the opening of a powder plant by DuPont in 1918. The city's population grew from 80,865 in 1900 to 110,364 in 1910 and would reach 118,342 by 1920. Added to the expanding population was September's Spanish influenza epidemic, in which 500,000 died nationwide. The existing institutions in 1918 were woefully inadequate to meet the growing medical needs of the community.

Chapter Two

PROTESTANT HOSPITAL

There will be no effort to operate the hospital for profit.
—1919 newspaper article on the
opening of Protestant Hospital

THE GROWTH OF NASHVILLE MEANT THAT THERE WAS a need for more hospitals, but no crisis had presented itself to push the citizenry into establishing them. The influenza epidemic changed that picture. Physicians ran out of hospital beds for patients. The public health argument was that physicians could treat more people and better isolate the epidemic through hospitalization rather than home treatment. Businessmen, physicians, lawyers, and clergymen responded to the crisis.

The names on the charter of incorporation for Protestant Hospital, December 12, 1918, were L. A. Bowers, Leslie Cheek, E. B. Craig, R. M. Dudley, and John A. Pitts. The founders bought property with existing buildings so that no time would be wasted in getting the hospital operational, and they had the foresight to buy plenty of land to allow for expansion. The sale of approximately $186,000 of fifteen-year 6 percent bonds, plus donations and gifts of citizens, made possible the purchase of the property and essential equipment and the improvement of buildings.

The plot of ten-and-a-half wooded acres consisted of two adjoining city blocks, generally referred to as the Murphy Home Place, bounded by four city streets: Church Street on the south, Twentieth Avenue on the east, Twenty-first Avenue on the west, and Patterson Street on the north. The widow of Samuel M. Murphy sold the property.

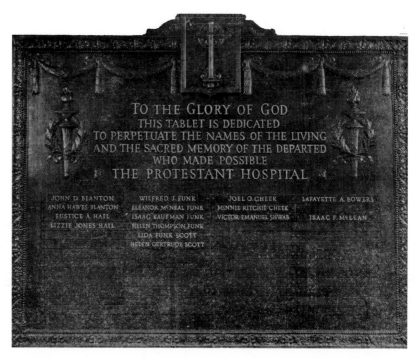

TO THE GLORY OF GOD
THIS TABLET IS DEDICATED
TO PERPETUATE THE NAMES OF THE LIVING
AND THE SACRED MEMORY OF THE DEPARTED
WHO MADE POSSIBLE
THE PROTESTANT HOSPITAL

JOHN D. BLANTON   WILFRED J. FUNK   JOEL O. CHEEK   LAFAYETTE A. BOWERS
ANNA HAWES BLANTON   ELEANOR McNEAL FUNK   MINNIE RITCHIE CHEEK
EUSTICE A. HAIL   ISAAC KAUFMAN FUNK   VICTOR EMANUEL SHWAB   ISAAC F. McLEAN
LIZZIE JONES HAIL   HELEN THOMPSON FUNK
                         LIDA FUNK SCOTT
                         HELEN GERTRUDE SCOTT

This plaque commemorates some of the dedicated people who worked together to make possible the existence of Protestant Hospital.

The land was originally part of a 640–acre grant awarded in 1784 by an act of the North Carolina Assembly to the pioneers who signed the Cumberland Compact, including Mark Robinson, John Boyd, and John Cockrill. In 1857 the Boyd property was divided among Boyd's heirs: Sarah Elizabeth, wife of John H. Williams; Mary Lemira, wife of Henry Martyn Hayes; Rachel Douglass, wife of Robert Smiley and, following his death, wife of Henry S. Foote, former governor of Mississippi; and John Overton Ewing, son of Major Boyd's wife, Lemira A. Douglass. Boyd Avenue, Douglass Avenue, and Hayes Street were named for these family members.

West of the Boyd property was a tract consisting of 360 acres originally acquired in 1816 by Joseph T. Elliston. And west of that property were 378 acres known as the Cockrill Spring tract, which was also owned by Major Boyd.

In 1869 and 1871 Samuel M. Murphy bought portions of the Boyd and Elliston estates, and he built a country estate surrounded by trees. Murphy, a millionaire recognized as Nashville's wealthiest citizen, was a whiskey distiller from Cincinnati who had made his fortune during the Civil War and had married Anna Hayes. Murphy died December 23, 1900.

The two major buildings on the Murphy property, which were to become the first two buildings of the Protestant Hospital complex, were the mansion (which at the time was the home of the Nashville College for Young Women, previously known as Buford College for Young Women, and before that as Ward's Seminary for Young Ladies) and the West Building (erected in 1900, also owned by the college).

The Murphy mansion became a dormitory for nurses in training, and the larger West Building was remodeled for $75,000 and converted into the hospital. It had eighty beds, a fully equipped surgical department, X-ray equipment, bacteriological and pathological labs, and maintenance facilities. Protestant Hospital received its name to distinguish it from Saint Thomas Hospital across Church Street, a Roman Catholic institution.

Protestant Hospital opened its doors on March 20, 1919. A newspaper article about the new hospital noted,

> An unusual feature of the management of the institution will be that the Protestant churches of the city will have an equal voice in the management. . . . It has been decided that no physician will be named on the board of governors, either now or in the future.
>
> The hospital is the outgrowth of a plan of the Ministers' Alliance of Nashville, and although under strong church influence, the hospital will be undenominational in its control.

The hospital was to take paying patients as well as charity patients. Nashvillians donated money to the hospital, and an engraved plaque in the lobby honored major benefactors. It read, "To the Glory of God this tablet is dedicated to perpetuate the names of the living and the sacred memory of the departed who made possible The Protestant Hospital." Names listed were Anna Hawes Blanton, John D. Blanton, Lafayette A. Bowers, Joel O. Cheek, Minnie Ritchie Cheek, Eleanor McNeal Funk, Helen Thompson Funk, Isaac

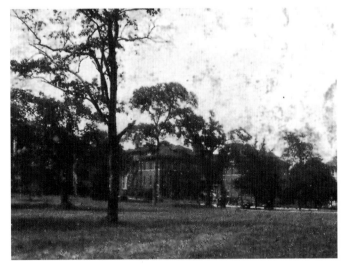

Protestant Hospital sat on ten-and-a-half wooded acres; the hospital site was bounded by four city streets: Church Street on the south, Twentieth Avenue on the east, Twenty-first Avenue on the west, and Patterson Street on the north.

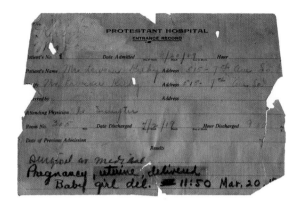

This entrance record is for Protestant Hospital's first patient, Anita Kilby.

Kaufman Funk, Wilfred J. Funk, Eustice A. Hail, Lizzie Jones Hail, Isaac F. McLean, Helen Gertrude Scott, Lida Funk Scott, and Victor Emanuel Shwab.

Protestant's first patient arrived on opening day. Gladys Kilby gave birth to a baby girl, Anita. Mother and child were discharged on April 2, 1919, thirteen days later. Anita Kilby Lewis would grow up to become a critical care nurse at Metro General Hospital, and Baptist Hospital would hold a special birthday party for her at the Women's Pavilion in 1998. Dr. T. G. Pollard was the attending physician. He was ninety-one years old in 1967 when the building in which Mrs. Lewis was born (then known as the West Building in the Baptist Hospital complex) was torn down to make way for a new one, and he participated in the celebration.

The first administrator at Protestant was Evander M. Sanders, M.D., a surgeon, who served until 1932. In that year he had to have emergency surgery for an "abdominal ailment" and was in the hospital at the time of his death. He survived the operation but knew it was a fatal illness. "He continued to direct various details of the institution until forbidden by his physicians," according to his obituary. A member of the American Medical Association, the Tennessee State Medical Association, the Nashville Academy of Medicine, the Southern Medical Association, the Davidson County Medical Society, and the Northwestern Surgical Association, Sanders was fifty-six years old when he died. The first superintendent was E. M. Fuqua; H. H. Campbell was secretary, and W. R. Wills was treasurer.

The other administrators of Protestant Hospital were V. I. Witherspoon (1933–37), Elizabeth Sloo (1937–45), and Lois B. Stow (1945–48), who had been assistant to Miss Sloo.

Some of the physicians at Protestant Hospital were Dr. W. A. Bryan, Dr. O. N. Bryan, Dr. Harrison Shoulders, Dr. J. T. Ross, Dr. Robert Grizzard, Dr. Tom Grizzard, Dr. Charles Brower, Dr. Rogers Herbert, Dr. Hettie Shoulders, and Dr. Frank Fessey. Many young physicians came back to Nashville after World War I, including Dr. George Carpenter, Dr. Paul Warner, and Dr. Sumpter Anderson.

In the first year of operation, there were 2,233 patients; 1,685 of them had major surgery and 65 had minor surgery. The hospital was so crowded that patients filled the sun parlors and virtually all other spaces. People had to be turned away, especially when a second influenza epidemic struck. The operation costs were $110,136.22, which included $18,933 in interest and discount payments on bonds and notes. The loss for the year was $2,792.30. The bulk of the income, $96,385, came from payments of patients. Inside payroll cost was $14,466, and administrators' payroll was $6,603. Other costs included $1,643 for insurance and $2,288 for the pharmacy. This optimistic statement appeared in the financial summary of the first year: "Considering the fact that the hospital was subject to the expenses of upkeep and carrying charges of the property for nearly a year before it began to receive any revenue, this is a splendid showing for the first year of work and a demonstration of the fact that with additional facilities now needed for the accommodation of more patients, the institution will be put on an earning basis that will enable it in a few years to retire all of its outstanding obligations." The optimism proved to be ill-founded.

The official number of births in Nashville for 1919 was 2,314; ten years later, it rose to 3,363. In 1920, Protestant Hospital welcomed the births of 105 babies.

The entire budget for 1922 was about $120,000. The hospital had 2,249 patients, which included 1,795 surgical patients and 39 babies. Protestant hospital's building program was modest but added to the community's growth toward a regional healthcare center. The East Building, completed in 1924, increased capacity to 210 beds and 18 bassinets. Nashville General Hospital had received a new charter and

"People are continually complaining about hospitals which is a little hard for me to understand. Now I am continually singing the praises of Baptist Hospital."
—Milbrey Luton

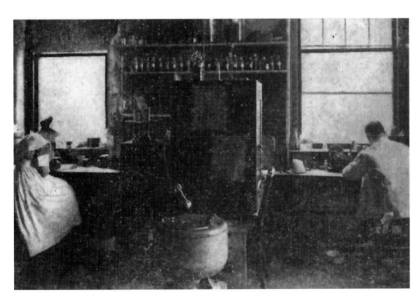

Protestant Hospital boasted its own laboratory facilities.

board in 1921, and in 1932 it would add a wing to increase its capacity from 65 to 260 patients.

The health of Nashvillians continued to be threatened by serious illnesses. From 1919 to 1929, the major reported communicable diseases in Nashville were typhoid and paratyphoid fever, diphtheria, scarlet fever, measles, and whooping cough, according to the city's health officer. The 1928 Tennessee State Health Department Vital Statistics Bulletin listed the major causes of death in Nashville: heart diseases, tuberculosis, apoplexy, chronic nephritis, cancer, pneumonia, influenza, other external causes, bronchopneumonia, and congenital conditions.

The Great Depression and Protestant's generally poor financial condition meant no more growth. The hospital went into receivership in 1932. Outstanding bonded indebtedness was $347,000, creditors were owed $40,000, and salaries were $1,100. Charles Nelson, president of Nashville Trust Company, was the receiver.

Nevertheless, the hospital continued its operation. In 1936, 3,234 patients were treated and 390 babies were born. By 1937, other infirmaries and hospitals had merged with Protestant Hospital, including Fort's Infirmary, Trinity Hospital, and the old Baptist Hospital, which was located at Eighth and Union Streets (the site of the present-day Federal Reserve Bank).

Several measures improved the hospital's efficiency. Around 1937 the X-ray department had a Kelly Ket Techron machine. The hospital made its own electricity and could draw on the power company, if necessary. It made its own ice and had cold storage for food. It also had a laundry.

Although Protestant Hospital received an "approved" rating from the Hospital Standardization Conference in 1940, its financial woes were unrelenting. In 1941, a bondholders committee repurchased the property at a cost of about $100,000 in an auction ordered by the court to satisfy creditors. The hospital was needed for general purposes, but state leaders considered converting it to a state tuberculosis hospital. Nashville leaders—government, civic, business, and medical—got together and exerted enough pressure that the state leaders settled on a site elsewhere in the city for the TB hospital.

A longtime employee, Mary E. Sesler, started working as the cashier at the hospital in 1944, following graduation from high school. She said,

"My thanks to everyone at Baptist Hospital for making my stay a nice one—my doctor and all the nurses. thanks again—should I need to come again, it would be easy."

A grateful patient,
—Pauline Johnson

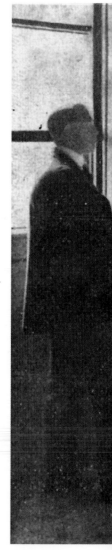

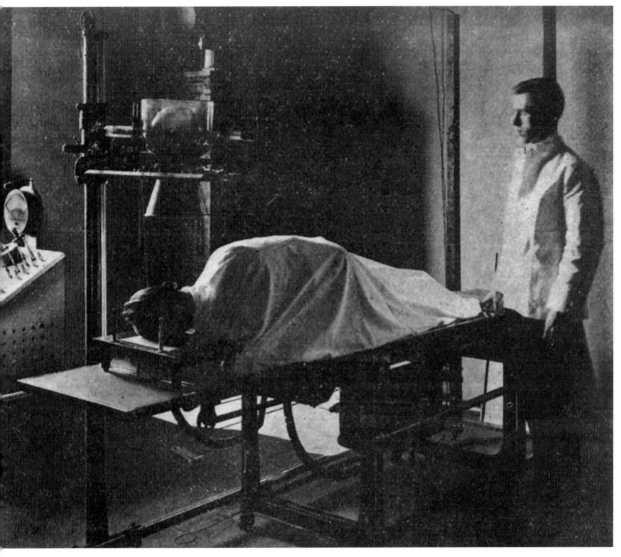

Even in its early days, Protestant Hospital had some specialized medical equipment, such as this X-ray equipment.

"All office employees were required to know how to relieve on the switchboard, admit and discharge patients, and do all other routine duties performed in the office." Sesler's primary duties included making the deposit each day and taking it to Nashville Bank and Trust Company downtown. Employees were paid in cash monthly, and part of the salary was a thirty-day cafeteria meal ticket. This practice continued until 1947 when Protestant started paying its employees by check.

Sesler described her work: "As cashier, it was my responsibility to post [by hand] all charges as they were brought to the Business Office each morning by the different departments. The cashier's office was open on weekends. At the end of each patient week, I would prepare a statement and take it to the patient's room. Hardly anyone had hospitalization insurance in those days, and bills were payable weekly. I can remember people signing notes for any unpaid balance."

Sesler added, "As a courtesy to the anesthesiologists and nurse anesthetists, the cashier collected their bills for them when the patient was dismissed from the hospital. The charge ranged from $10 to $15 to $20."

Some of the physicians she remembered seeing often at Protestant Hospital were Dr. T. G. Pollard, Dr. Robert Grizzard, Dr. Frank Fessey, Dr. John Cayce, Dr. Paul DeWitt, Dr. W. J. Core, Dr. A. B. Thatch Sr., Dr. Hugh Barr, Dr. J. C. Pennington, Dr. Roger Burrus, and Dr. Sumpter Anderson. Other physicians who practiced at the hospital after World War II were Dr. Elkin Rippy, Dr. Ray Fessey, Dr. Jim Hayes, Dr. Jim Kirtley, Dr. Cleo Miller, and Dr. Charles Trabue.

The hospital's financial statement had not improved over the years. Financial realities had outweighed the good intentions of the administrators in trying to keep costs low to better serve the public and had brought the hospital to the point of going into receivership on January 2, 1943, to Nashville Trust Company. By 1948 the hospital's debt stood at almost $500,000, and deterioration of the physical plant was becoming a serious problem. Protestant Hospital was in no shape—financial or otherwise—to meet the challenges posed by a postwar world. The hospital's future looked bleak indeed.

A bill for the birth of a baby gives some idea of hospital charges in the late 1930s.

Chapter Three

MID-STATE BAPTIST HOSPITAL

We learned how to operate a hospital with efficiency.
—Rev. Dr. James L. Sullivan

REV. DR. JAMES L. SULLIVAN STATED, "I WAS BACK IN MY study at Belmont Heights with my chin in my hands, thinking about [Protestant hospital's situation], and the door popped open. And Jack Massey came in and I could tell how excited he was. He said, 'I just learned that Protestant Hospital is going bankrupt.' And I said, 'Well, thank the Lord!' He said, 'Don't thank Him till you find out what the facts were. They've just bought $40,000 worth of equipment from me, and I can't stand that kind of loss. It's going to throw me into bankruptcy.' I said, 'Well, they've got just exactly what we need for a Baptist hospital and it affords an opportunity and I think I see a way out for you to get your $40,000 and for us to get a hospital in the same deal.' He said, 'You think we could do this?' And I said, 'I know we can.'" And they did.

Sullivan, a native Mississippian, attended Mississippi College before entering the seminary. He became the pastor at Belmont Heights Baptist Church in 1946. He also became executive secretary (chief executive officer) for the Baptist Sunday School Board in 1946, a job he held for many years.

He felt that "hospitals are to a denomination what a fortress is to the military. My deep interest in hospitals came when I was in Mississippi and they needed to double the size of the Baptist Hospital and I led in the movement. We succeeded in getting funds and building the hospital just before coming to Nashville. My background experience had made me almost fanatical in my support of our Baptist hospitals." He was certainly a strong force in establishing Nashville's Mid-State Baptist Hospital.

Massey, born in Sandersville, Georgia, and reared there and in Macon, went to the University of Florida. Then he became manager of a drugstore, Liggett Drugs, where he worked with an uncle, Alec Brown. In 1929, Massey was asked to manage the Liggett Drug Company on Church Street in Nashville. He later established the Massey Surgical Supply Company, and that company was the one endangered by the precarious financial status of Protestant Hospital.

Sullivan recalled that Massey "proposed the possibility of our getting enough interested men together to see if we could effect a transfer of the institution into Baptist management. Sensing the importance of this move, we acted without delay."

Sullivan and Massey divided the tasks that led to the transfer of the hospital's ownership. He urged Massey to "take the responsibility of making contact with the creditors. You are one of them and can assure

The delivery room was—and still remains—an integral part of the hospital's services to the community. However, present-day delivery rooms no longer look as uninviting as this one.

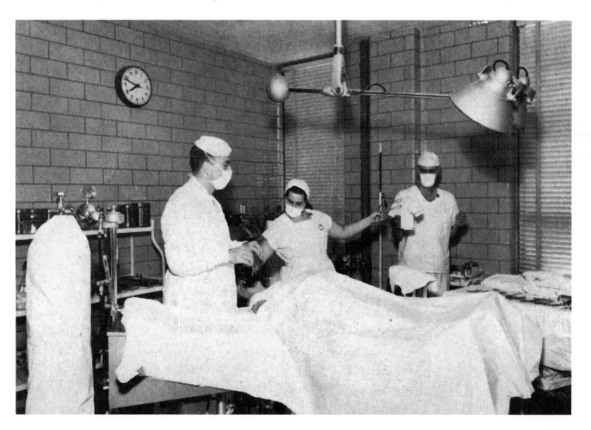

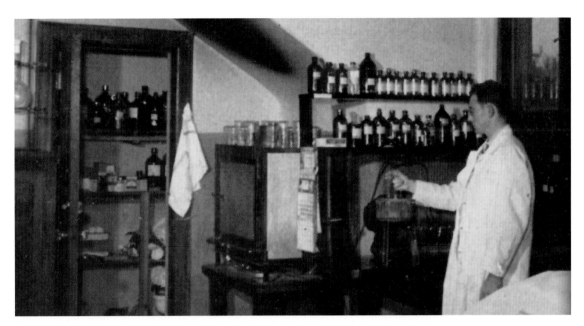

The clinical laboratory played a major role in the hospital. The equipment may have changed over the years, but the integral role has not.

them that if they will give us a few months, three at the most, we believe with all of our hearts that we can pay them back in full or at least sign a contract with them that is binding that we will pay back every penny that we owe them with interest. . . . Also you should make contact with the chairman of the self-perpetuating board of trustees of the Protestant Hospital to see if he would be willing to work with us to try to transfer ownership into Baptists' hands so we can operate it as a denominational institution."

Massey was also to contact a lawyer to find out how to transfer the property legally from the board to the Baptists. He was the man for the job. According to his daughter, Barbara Massey Rogers, "Daddy could bring people together and make them compromise on both sides and make things happen." She added, "One of the things I admire—and he never lost this touch—was that he enjoyed knowing the nurses, he enjoyed knowing the doctors, he enjoyed knowing the janitors. He never lost the common touch. It started back when he was associated with Baptist, and he had it the day he died at Good Samaritan Hospital in Palm Beach, Florida."

Sullivan's tasks were to contact Dr. C. W. Pope, executive secretary of the Tennessee Baptist Convention, to see how he would feel about the project; suggest a new organizational structure for the hospital to make transition to Baptists smooth; and submit a list of Baptists who might accept the responsibility of rescuing Protestant Hospital.

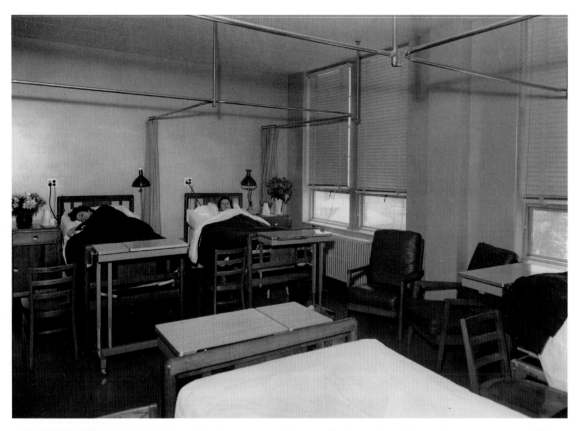

Sharing rooms was the rule rather than the exception at Mid-State Baptist Hospital and other hospitals; private rooms were not the norm until the latter part of the twentieth century.

Pope was in favor of the idea, but the Tennessee Baptist Convention had voted not to accept title to any property against which there was indebtedness. Sullivan noted that with the assistance of lawyers and others, they secured several Baptist men who, as individuals, were interested in seeing the hospital operated efficiently and effectively "for our Baptist people." The men would be personally responsible for the debt if the hospital could not become profitable. These names appear on the amended charter of Protestant Hospital to enact the transfer to Tennessee Baptists: Jack C. Massey, A. E. Batts, Albert B. Maloney, A. Roy Greene, Will Ed Gupton, Russell Brothers, Will T. Cheek, Chalmers Cowan, Martin S. Roberts, W. F. Powell, James L. Sullivan, G. Allen West, George B. Graves, W. L. Stigler, J. Harold Stephens, Andrew D. Tanner, and William Gupton. Sullivan clearly recognized, as he wrote in 1988, that it "could be expensive to us personally if the project failed. At the same time it held almost limitless potential for the future if we could make it succeed." They were getting only one building of any worth (and it was later torn down to make space for the Gene Kidd Building facing Twenty-first Avenue). The older buildings were dilapidated. Of course the property itself had value.

Sullivan described what happened: "On an agreed day the transfer was made. It was in this manner: one of the trustees of the Protestant Hospital would resign; then in turn one of our volunteers would be elected to take his place. This was done person by person until one group had resigned and another had been elected. After the last trustee of the Protestant Hospital had resigned and the last individual from our group of volunteers had been elected, the old trustees stood as a body, thanked us for taking so many headaches off their hands, and they walked from the room.

"The institution was ours.

"The new group of trustees organized themselves with Mr. Massey as chairman. Then they proceeded to elect a new manager of the hospital. Renovations and drastic internal reorganizations began immediately."

The Protestant Hospital was turned over without cost to the Tennessee Baptist Convention. They named it Mid-State Baptist Hospital because they were defining an area to serve, that is, between the mountains and the Tennessee River and the state lines. In April of 1948, the Executive Committee of the Tennessee Baptist Convention appointed a Board of Trustees, consisting of seventeen members, to supersede a like number of trustees, who at that time were operating the Protestant Hospital. On June 1, 1948, Robert M. Murphy became the hospital's administrator.

The members of the Board of Trustees of Protestant Hospital as of 1947 were R. Elmer Baulch, F. A. Berry, Homer Brown, A. M. Burton, Newman Cheek (secretary), C. A. Craig (chairman), Brownlee Currey, Lipscomb Davis, Bernard Fensterwald, F. E. Gillette (vice chairman), William Gupton, T. Graham Hall (chairman of the Executive Committee), Harry Howe, Warner McNeilly (assistant treasurer), Charles Nelson Jr., Walter Stokes Jr., and Joe Werthan (treasurer).

Joining Massey and Sullivan on the first board of Mid-State Baptist Hospital were Albert Maloney, Russell Brothers, Chalmers Cowan, G. Allen West, J. Harold Stephens, Andrew D. Tanner, A. E. Batts, W. L. Stigler, Will Ed Gupton, H. G. Bernard, Will T. Cheek, Hardin Conn, George B. Graves, A. Roy Greene, William Gupton, John W. Harton, George Pardue, W. F. Powell, Martin S. Roberts, and Roy Byrn. These men joined in November 1948: J. F. Brewer, J. C. Edgar, Stirton Oman, Howard Smith, Lem B. Stevens, and J. W. Zumbro.

"Being a business man, I know how difficult it is to run an efficient ship without losing the personal touch. You have done just that."
—Calvin Houghland

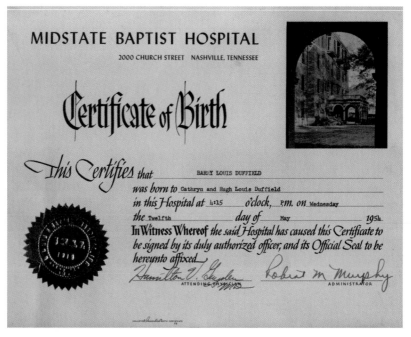

MIDSTATE BAPTIST HOSPITAL

2000 CHURCH STREET   NASHVILLE, TENNESSEE

Certificate of Birth

This Certifies that   BARRY LOUIS DUFFIELD

was born to Cathryn and Hugh Louis Duffield

in this Hospital at 4:15 *o'clock,* P.M. *on* Wednesday

the Twelfth *day of* May   1954

In Witness Whereof the said Hospital has caused this Certificate to be signed by its duly authorized officer, and its Official Seal to be hereunto affixed

ATTENDING PHYSICIAN   ADMINISTRATOR

The hospital has always been a community leader in the birth of babies. This elaborate birth certificate records the arrival of another one. The late Hugh Duffield worked at Baptist, as does his son Barry whose birth is recorded here.

An early question posed to the board was, "Are only Baptists to be served?" Sullivan remembered the board's response: "We said, 'No. It's going to be a ministry to humanity.' 'Well, what about all races?' 'Yes, sir!' It didn't matter what background or ethnic group. If they are in need, we minister to them and we do it at this place."

The board and Sullivan shared this philosophy about how the hospital should be run: "It ought to be done in a religious way, highly ethical. But it ought to be up to date, use modern methods. People deserve the best—all races, all people—and regardless of their cultural backgrounds, religious differences, there are similarities here in our desire to maintain health and live a long time."

Sullivan, who served several years on the board, summarized the board's approach to the newly acquired hospital: "We learned how to operate a hospital with efficiency and without raising prices, how to pay off debts, and how to build or accrue enough reserves to build your parking lots, your buildings, and this they have done from that day on."

Chapter 4

NURSES AND THE SCHOOL OF NURSING

We believe that man is a physical, mental, emotional, spiritual, and social being, whose health needs are ever changing within a changing society.
—First tenet of the philosophy of the Mid-State Baptist Hospital School of Nursing, 1959–61

PRIOR TO 1918, MOST NURSING EDUCATION WAS accomplished by physicians who set up small clinics and had schools of nursing associated with them. Several young women received training as they helped the physicians in return. Just as it needed more hospitals and more healthcare-related services, Nashville needed more nurses and efficient ways to train them.

The School of Nursing was one of Protestant hospital's most successful enterprises. It started on March 20, 1919, with nine students, who were accepted for "three years of uninterrupted application." The entrance requirements included having an eighth grade education and being at least sixteen years old. The number of students grew to forty-two by April 1920.

The young women—there were no young men!—had to furnish their own thermometers, prep trays, and scissors. Students worked twelve hours a day in addition to receiving their class instruction. They had a half

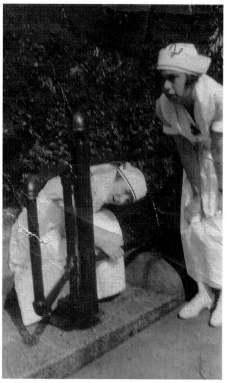

In 1920, two nursing students took a break from classes at the School of Nursing.

day off per week. Chapel, which was not affiliated with any specific denomination, was mandatory at 6:00 A.M. each day. Students lived in a dorm with six persons per room. No dating was allowed.

The students prepared food trays as a part of meeting patients' needs. By 1924, if not before, senior students were allowed to give medications. The pay scale was $6 per month for first-year students, $8 for second-year, and $10 for third-year.

Most courses were taught at the hospital, but students went to George Peabody College for Teachers to learn bacteriology, chemistry, and nutrition. The nursing of children was a three-month program at Cincinnati Children's Hospital.

A 1943 graduate of the school recalled that student nurses were required to fold dirty linen and remove it from the patient's room in a neat bundle. Nurses were required to stand when a doctor entered the room.

Following the U.S. entrance into World War II, the need for even more nurses intensified. The Nurse Training Act of 1943 provided for funds to institutions willing to offer an accelerated curriculum for the war effort. In that year 95 percent of nursing students in the country were in the U.S. Cadet Nurse Corps, and Protestant Hospital's school was accepted as a participant in the Corps. Students' allowances were $15 per month for the first nine months, then $20 per month for twenty-one months. The students also received outdoor summer and winter uniforms, indoor uniforms, and textbooks. They had to agree to "stay in essential nursing, civilian or military, for the duration of the war emergency." They became registered nurses after passing a state exam. The Corps ended in 1945, but classes funded by the act continued until 1948. Records for 1946 indicate that young women needed to be in good health, be eighteen to thirty-five years old, and have a high school education to enter the school.

Edith Good, Grace Anderson, Pauline Thompson, Pat Manning, and Nellie Griffin were among the nursing staff at Protestant Hospital. In its final years as Protestant Hospital School of Nursing, the school's director was Mary D. Ross. Rev. Prentice A. Pugh was the chaplain, and the instructors included Naomi Bingham Matthews, Virginia Woeller Racker, Gladys Stone, Clara R. Greene, Lily Lane McCorkle, Mary Elizabeth Ingraham, Leta Whitley, Ernestine Martin Ralls, Marie Medford, Mary Fuller Smith, Muriel Pennington, Edna Earle Hickey, Calysta Jeankins, and Lura Vaughn Murray. Some of the physicians who gave supplementary lectures were Dr. J. J. Ashby, Dr. J. S. Cayce, Dr. J. I. Fuqua, Dr. J. C. Pennington, Dr. W. W. Wilkerson Jr., and Dr. R. E. Wyatt.

The Mid-State Baptist Hospital, Inc., School of Nursing was organized in June 1948 following the dissolution of the original school at the time of the hospital's new relationship with the Tennessee Baptist Convention. In the early 1950s the students were the evening and night shift staff except for a shift supervisor. Among their duties were mixing IVs, preparing diet trays for the patients, and going to the basement to retrieve oxygen tanks. The primary drug was penicillin. Many students recalled that in surgery, the windows would be open with the fans going in the summertime. There was no recovery room.

"Thanks is no way a complete comment for how I feel toward Baptist hospital and staff. It's been my 'mis' fortune of being in several hospitals in my life, but none even approach Baptist in any way. From pre-surgery diagnostics to admission (EMA), through surgery to the care afterwards in my room, it was absolutely top flight. I pray that God continue to work miracles there with the best hospital and staff in the world."

—James Mills

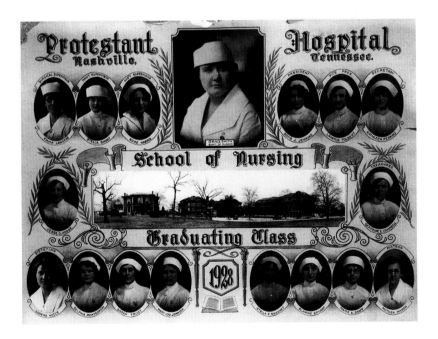

These students graduated from Protestant Hospital's School of Nursing in 1928.

Nashville was home to six accredited schools of nursing in 1951: Madison Sanitarium, Saint Thomas, General, Vanderbilt, Mid-State Baptist, and Meharry Medical. The general courses were the same, but Vanderbilt's and Meharry's were considered collegiate programs. This point became even more significant in coming years to the future of the hospital-related nursing schools, called diploma programs.

A new five-story School of Nursing was completed and occupied in 1956. It had facilities for 175 nurses. The Tennessee Board of Nursing and National League for Nursing accredited the $1 million school. The school subsidized student nurses over and above the tuition they paid and credit allowed for their service.

Students came from across the region to attend the nursing school, and at least two came from across the world: both Huo Mei Ling from Siba, Sarawak, Borneo, and Glaphré Kay Spencer from Swaziland, South Africa, were present in the early 1960s.

Specialized nurses' training in cardiac care came about through a two-day symposium in 1969. The attendance by four hundred nurses pointed to the interest in the topic. Janie Sullivan, one of the Directors of Nurses, attributed the success of this and other cardiac programs to Dr. Fred Ownby.

The Baptist School of Nursing closed in 1970. William Johnson was then serving as Director of Nurses. He was in the unique position

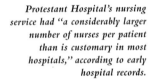

Protestant Hospital's nursing service had "a considerably larger number of nurses per patient than is customary in most hospitals," according to early hospital records.

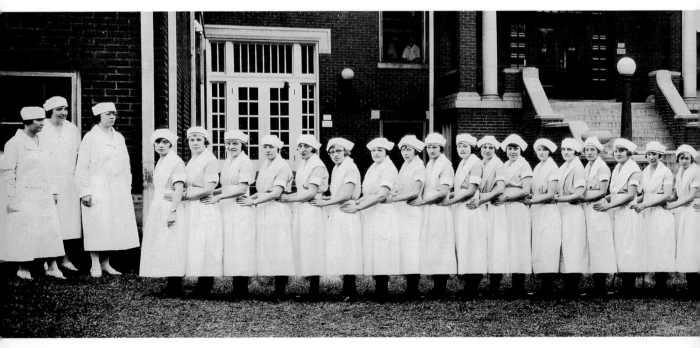

of having been a male registered nurse at a time when few men went into the profession and then going on to become a member of the hospital's administrative staff. He explained why the school was closed: "Nurses upon graduation were not staying with us and helping us. They were going elsewhere to places that had not contributed anything to nursing. Consequently, we felt that was not a wise use of our money, and secondly, the National League for Nursing, which was the accredited body for nursing education, had come out and said that within so many years all nurses that are considered professional nurses will go to universities of higher learning for degrees."

He added that nurses "were striving to be recognized as a profession and professional people do not get it in hospital nursing programs—you go to universities to get that. So, we thought we saw the writing on the wall and we decided to get out of nursing education."

From the time the school opened in 1919 until it closed in 1970, there were 1,038 graduates. The smallest class was in 1935 with four graduates, a statistic that is hardly surprising given the wide-ranging effects of the Great Depression on society. The largest class was in 1964 with 46 graduates; many years in the 1960s had graduating classes of 30 to 40 members.

Baptist Hospital briefly operated a school to train licensed practical nurses. For example, in 1994 about fifty students participated at a cost

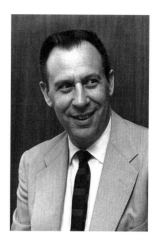

William Johnson, who began his career as a registered nurse at a time when few males went into the profession, went on to become Director of Nurses and later Senior Vice President of Professional Affairs.

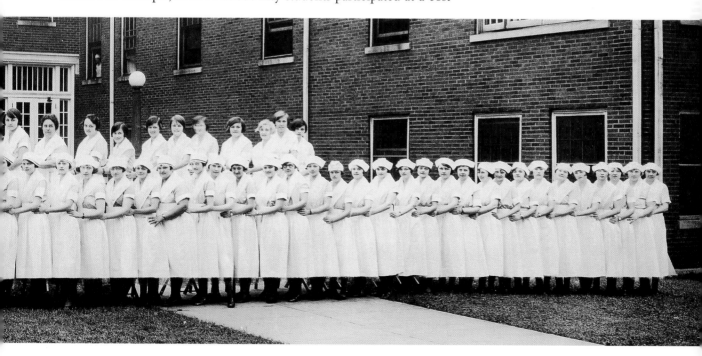

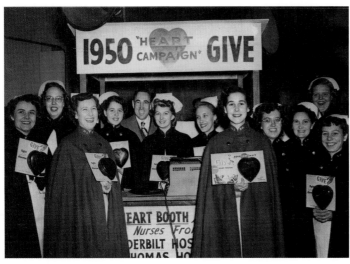

A 1950 Heart Campaign in the community gained support from nursing students.

of $300,000 to the hospital.

Janie Sullivan, whose training history included General Hospital, Peabody for a B.S.N., and Vanderbilt for an M.A., was an instructor in the nursing school beginning in 1953, became the Director of Nursing Education from 1959 to 1968, and then became the Director of the School of Nursing from 1971 to 1976. At one time she was responsible for seven hundred employees in Nursing Service, the largest department in the hospital.

Sullivan noted the differences between nurses who had been through a diploma program and those who had been through a collegiate program. Students in the diploma programs received more clinical experience from the beginning of their training. After she had spent three months in a diploma program, long before her graduation, she was in charge of a unit under the supervision of one RN.

Sullivan recently experienced nursing care as a patient at Baptist Hospital, which she considered "excellent." Nurses now take heart and lung sounds, but nurses were not permitted to do that only a few years ago. And they were told in the early years that cardiopulmonary

The Alphonso H. Bean Employee Memorial plaque reads in part, "In honor of Alphonso H. Bean, healing nurse, patient advocate and loving mentor. With more than 23 years of service to patients at Baptist Hospital, Mrs. Bean exemplified the commitment and dedication to patients and their care that so ⸱⸱⸱ ⸱⸱y Baptist employees bring to our institution."

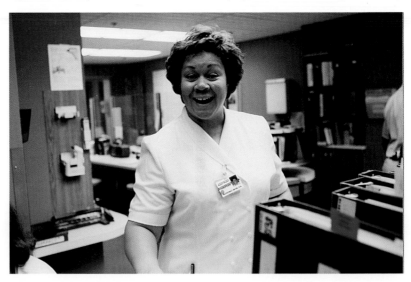

resuscitation (CPR) was dangerous because a patient's ribs could be fractured. Sullivan pointed out that having fractured ribs as a result of CPR or dying because CPR was not administered was not much of a choice.

According to Sullivan, nursing students lived in three different buildings at Baptist Hospital, each with a house mother. Classes were held downstairs in each. The West Building was the School of Nursing. A house mother was on duty at all times, and only students, parents, and the housekeeping staff were allowed upstairs. Students had to be in the dorm by 10:30 or 11:00 P.M. Discipline for infractions of the rules included being campused for a certain period of time. House mothers had keys to all rooms and all lockers and the right to use them. No alcohol was allowed. In return for a scholarship, a student had to work at Baptist about one year in return. The National League for Nursing set standards for schools, and Baptist's had approval.

It was "satisfying to work in the School of Nursing, no matter what the position. So many students have gone on and done well. It's good to hear from former students," said Sullivan. During her time on the administrative staff, occupancy was 85 to 90 percent. There were nursing shortages in many years, and all hospitals had difficulty getting and keeping enough RNs. Evelyn Springer, currently the Senior Vice President for Patient Care Services, has observed that there seems to be a cycle with a nursing shortage about every ten years.

"They pampered me at Baptist Hospital. The nurse even called me after I went home to make sure I was okay."

—Dale Haworth

Sullivan remarked on the hospital's growth under the leadership of Gene Kidd: "He was a good administrator; he was understanding of people; he had no difficulty making decisions. He was so organized that there was rarely a paper clip on his desk."

Addie Hamilton was Vice President and Night Administrator of Nursing Service at the time of her retirement in 1994. She trained at Nashville's General Hospital School of Nursing, Peabody/Vanderbilt, and Frontier Nursing in Windover, Kentucky. She began working at Baptist in 1960.

When she started, "patients weren't as sick nor were there advances in computers or machines, so you did not have to deal with those." Nurses have more responsibility, and they need more skills today.

Evelyn Springer came to Baptist Hospital in 1965 to go to the nursing program and graduated in 1968 and has been there ever since. She started on the night shift on the orthopedic unit, worked her way up to a head nurse position on the orthopedic unit, and became a supervisor. She then became what is known as a clinical director. While she was a clinical director she was also going back to school part-time to work on her Bachelor of Science in Nursing, and then when she

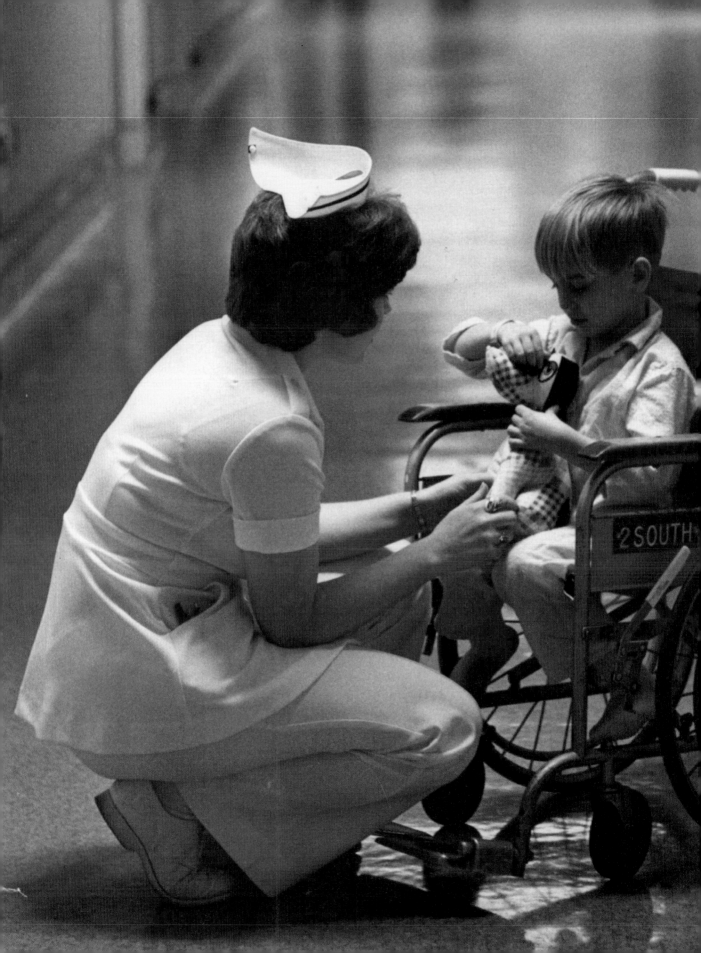

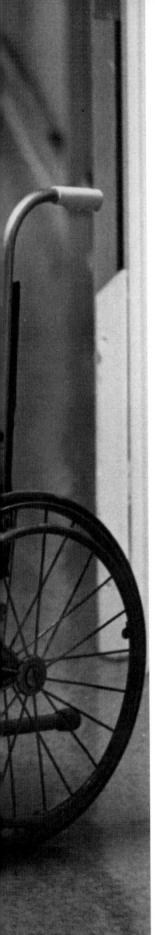

completed that in August of 1980. After receiving her BSN in 1980, she took a leave of absence and went to Vanderbilt University to do graduate work in nursing where she received her Master of Science degree in nursing. She came back to Baptist in 1982 and assumed the position of Vice President in Nursing. Two years later she was promoted to Senior Vice President. In addition, Springer serves on the Tennessee Board of Nursing. She was appointed to her first term by Governor Ned McWherter and to her second term by Governor Don Sundquist. She is currently serving as Chairman of that board. David Stringfield commented about her, "Evelyn Springer has truly come through the ranks to be the finest director of nursing that Baptist Hospital has had. She is truly a dedicated person whose interest has always been to put the patient first in every consideration. Due to her leadership and the efforts of all employees at Baptist Hospital, the community recognizes the hospital as the most caring and friendly facility by a wide margin compared to other hospitals in the region."

Springer's desire to become a nurse went back to her childhood. Many nurses likely share that with her. Her mother was a registered nurse whom she always admired and respected. As a child, Springer saw her mother being sought out by family and friends for healthcare advice and she also witnessed her mother assisting whenever a crisis situation occurred. This inspired Springer to become a nurse.

After the initial closing of its nursing school, "Baptist very heavily funded Belmont's nursing program when they were a two-year program. Most of those two-year programs have now gone to the four-year bachelor programs, but there are a few two-year programs," said Springer. There are several educational avenues to become a nurse: the two-year associate degree, three-year diploma programs, four-year BSN programs, or a masters program. All require passing scores on the state examination for registered nurse.

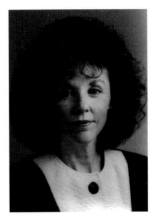

Evelyn Springer is currently the Senior Vice President for Patient Care Services; she has been a registered nurse at Baptist Hospital for thirty years.

Left:
A pediatric patient receives personal attention, a goal of all Baptist Hospital nurses.

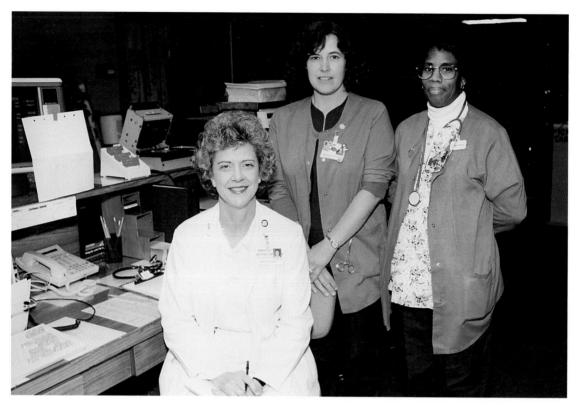

Patient surveys always acknowledge the caring and friendly attitude of nurses at Baptist Hospital. Left to right, Betty Cordell, RN, Brenda Dotson RN, and Deadra Hall, RN, are three good examples of this attitude.

Prior to 1960 there were very few male nurses. When two male nurses graduated from Baptist's nursing school in 1961, it left only one male student in the nursing school. Today more men are entering the field. Almost 8 percent of nurses in the state of Tennessee, for example, now are male.

Springer is confident about the past and future dedication of nurses: "Everybody said all the nurses will walk out when you start dealing with AIDS. . . . Nurses aren't going to walk out. Nurses have dealt with life-threatening illnesses throughout the history of mankind."

Particularly since 1980, Baptist Hospital has had remarkable expansion in the number of buildings, and Springer and the nurses have been able to offer their input: "If you're going to build a hospital, you need to ask a nurse how to build it because she's the one who's going to work there. . . . Those have been interesting programs—to become involved in the building of the hospital, to make it efficient, to make it better for patients. Nurses' contributions to such projects have proved invaluable to Baptist Hospital."

What did she foresee for the future of nursing? Springer said, "Baptist has never had a problem with staying on the cutting edge or keeping ahead or having the vision to see where we should be going or what we should be doing. I think leadership in nursing is going to be very challenging in the future, considering the vast changes in health care."

Technological advances are exciting and are "to be embraced" so that nurses can spend more time nursing. Springer emphasized that any change that can increase the nurse's time with the patient is positive. More computers are inevitable; a paperless routine with no charts would streamline steps. Most nurses now in Baptist Hospital have a wireless phone, and the patient knows the nurse's name and the extension number on each shift. "This has been a very valuable use of technology," Springer said, "improving communication for the nurse and for the patient."

Patients should expect quality care when they enter a hospital. As a rule, patients are much sicker today than even twenty years ago; the hospital is becoming a place primarily for the seriously ill. When it was first done at Baptist, a total hip replacement was a new procedure requiring a two-week hospital stay. Now the patient has surgery the first day, and the stay is about four days. Nurses have a harder time bonding with patients now because of abbreviated hospital stays and because of the severity of their patients' condition.

Nurses are likely to become more mobile as it becomes easier to be licensed nationwide, rather than on a state-by-state basis. With the aging of the baby boomers a much greater need for geriatric care in various stages seems more than likely. Nurses may also go into more fields in the community. Presently most registered nurses in Tennessee work in some capacity in hospitals.

Nursing has changed in many ways since 1919 and is more than likely to continue to change in the future. One thing is certain, however. The nursing staff at Baptist Hospital will continue to be dedicated to the patients "whose health needs are ever changing within a changing society."

"From my surgeon—to the nursing staff—the Rehabilitation Center and its personnel—the home care followup—all the way down to your housekeeping and maintenance personnel, I have never before been looked after and cared for as thoroughly and respectfully and kindly."

—Helen Pazienza

Superintendents of Nursing and Directors of Nurses
In the 1940s the name of the position changed to Director. There are some overlaps in years because of an individual's partial-year service. Existing records do not cite first names of some persons.

1919	Miss Busy
1919–20	Miss Bent
1920	Miss Hargis
1920–21	Miss Nichol
1921	Mrs. Rice
1921–23	Miss Moore
1923–28	Miss Grace Smith
1928	Miss Margaret Chesmire
1928–29	Miss Emma B. Landers
1929–30	Miss Rose Thelma Harris
1930	Mrs. Dot Smallwood
1930–32	Miss Edith Good
1932–33	Miss Elizabeth Proctor
1933–37	Miss Elizabeth Sloo
1937–41	Miss Helen Peterson
1941–43	Miss Elmelia Wellman
1943	Miss Louise Lillie Glasgow
1943–45	Miss Nina D. Gage
1946	Miss Mary D. Ross
1946–47	Mrs. Naomi B. Matthews
1947–48	Mrs. Virginia Racker
1948–54	Miss Grace Behrens
1954–55	Miss Carolyn Quigley
1955–57	Miss Lynn W. Bertholf
1958–59	Miss Margie Janssen
1959–67	Mrs. Lura Murray
1968–71	Mr. William Johnson
1971–76	Mrs. Janie Sullivan
1976–80	Mr. William Johnson
1981–	Evelyn Smith Springer

Directors of Nursing Education
1956–57	Nancy Travis
1958–59	Lessie Pride
1959–68	Janie Sullivan

Chapter 5

MANAGEMENT AND ADMINISTRATION

Baptist Hospital is a team effort.
—C. David Stringfield
President and CEO, Baptist Hospital

BEGINNING IN JUNE OF 1948, THE BOARD OF TRUSTEES and the administrative staff implemented many positive changes, such as renovating and reequipping the existing buildings, employing a full-time pathologist and anesthesiologist, hiring a chaplain to plan a religious program, updating the nursing service, and instituting a sound financial program of operation. The hospital cared for more and more patients. Mid-State Baptist Hospital (renamed simply Baptist Hospital in 1964) was on its way to becoming one of the leading hospitals in the state and, in fact, a healthcare provider to people from southern Kentucky and northern Alabama as well as Middle Tennessee. The role of all of the administrators and boards in moving the hospital forward to its prominent position in 1998 cannot be overemphasized.

Robert M. Murphy served as administrator from 1948 to 1953 with the assistance of Jamie Cheek as bookkeeper. When Murphy resigned, Terry Hiers Jr. oversaw the hospital temporarily until the arrival of Gene Kidd on June 13, 1954.

Kidd was a native of Petersburg, Virginia, who had attended William and Mary College and Washington and Lee University. Then he did administrative work in military hospitals while in the U.S. Air

Force during World War II. Before coming to Baptist, Kidd was the administrator of Phoebe Putney Memorial Hospital in Albany, Georgia. His first assistant was Terry Hiers Jr., followed by Robert P. Brueck, Barry Spero, and David Stringfield. Kidd assumed the title of executive director of Baptist Hospital in 1966, then became president in 1970 and served until 1981 at which time he became president emeritus. He was a Fellow in the American College of Hospital Administrators and had been its chairman; he was president of the Tennessee Hospital Association at one time; and he was a member of the Tennessee Board of Nursing for ten years.

Kidd's first secretary was Dorothy Barry. Then Mary Sesler was asked to fill the vacancy in 1958, and Irma Pardon eventually made it a two-secretary office. Sesler remembered, "It has been such a challenge working as a secretary to Mr. Kidd and watching the hospital grow under his leadership—whether it was picking up the morning mail or typing a paper for him as chairman of the American College of Hospital Administrators [ACHA] to deliver to the Australian Institute of Hospital Administration 1973 Congress in Adelaide, Australia, when he traveled around the world visiting healthcare facilities and evaluating the systems of the many countries!

"It was exciting to observe as Mr. Kidd served on the many committees and especially the many committees of the ACHA. Long

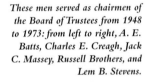

These men served as chairmen of the Board of Trustees from 1948 to 1973: from left to right, A. E. Batts, Charles E. Creagh, Jack C. Massey, Russell Brothers, and Lem B. Stevens.

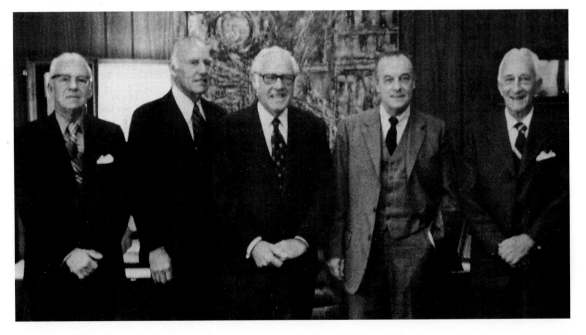

before he became chairman of the ACHA, I remarked to Irma [Pardon] one day, 'Irma, you just watch it. He's going to be chairman of the college one day.' I was right! One of my most thrilling moments came when I witnessed the dedication of the new hospital wing in his name—the Gene Kidd Building. I have seen many people seek his counsel and guidance.

"I remember so well the trustees and the Executive Committee of the Board of Trustees of the hospital—meeting and getting to know so many of these fine people over the years."

Jack Massey, Dr. Allen West, and Al Batts recruited Kidd for the job at Mid-State Baptist; Massey had met him at the Southern Hospital meetings. Kidd commented that it was an old hospital, and "we knew it was going to take money and we didn't have any money, so it was going to have to be a strong effort on the part of the medical staff, the Board of Trustees, and the administration. It was a triad that we started working with, and it was the best thing that ever happened to me."

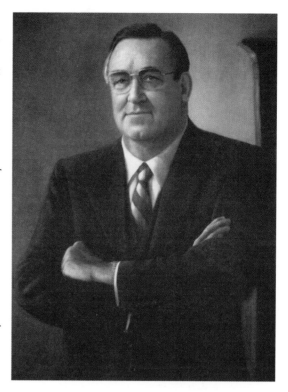

Gene Kidd was hired as the hospital's administrator in 1954; he retired in 1981 as president emeritus.

Kidd continued, "There were two men in my opinion totally responsible for Baptist Hospital being here—Jack Massey and Dr. James Sullivan." He also mentioned favorably the contributions of Dr. Charles C. Trabue, Dr. George Carpenter, Dr. Bob McCracken, Dr. Jim Thomasson, Albert Maloney, Russell Brothers, and Chalmers Cowan.

Kidd was very proud that the hospital "didn't borrow a dollar, never owed a dollar. That was because of this triad I had working with me. I didn't have a lot of doctors who were begging for equipment we couldn't afford. We would build as we went along." The timely purchase of land was a wise move too.

Under Kidd's leadership, Baptist Hospital grew from 210 beds to 724 beds, Middle Tennessee's largest healthcare facility.

C. David Stringfield succeeded Gene Kidd as president of Baptist in 1982. He is a native of Nashville. He received his master's degree in school administration from Peabody and his master's degree in hospital administration from Washington University. He did his residency at

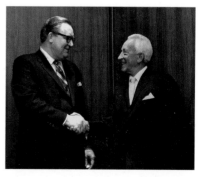

Gene Kidd and Lem B. Stevens, who was chairman of the board, share a congratulatory moment.

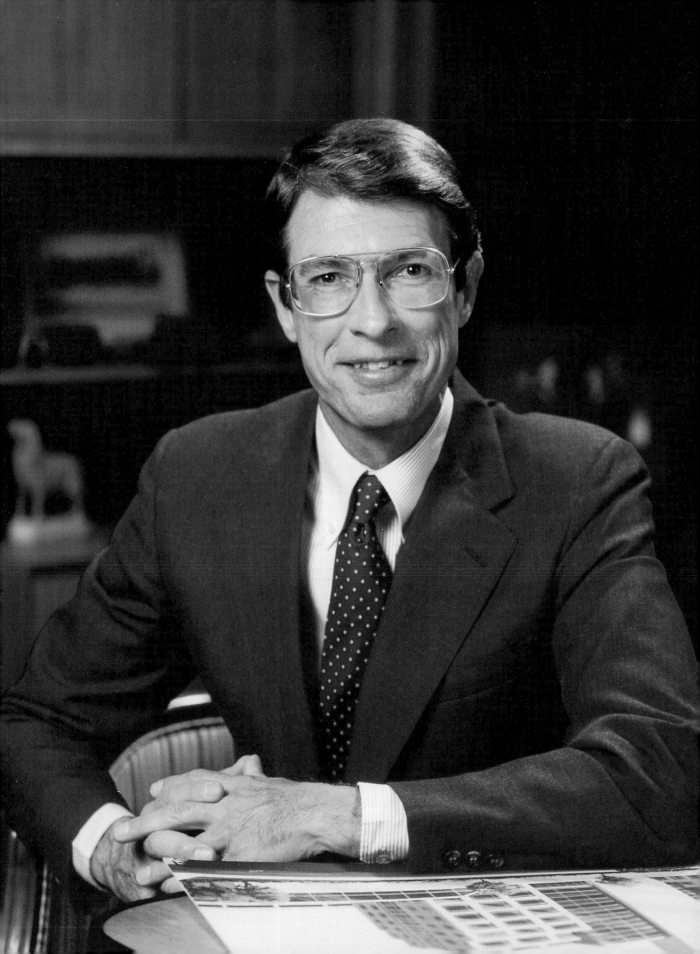

Milwaukee County General Hospital, then became assistant director of the Tennessee Hospital Association (1966–68) and executive director of the Tennessee Nursing Home Association (1966–67). His first position at Baptist was administrative director in 1968. Next he became executive vice president and chief operating officer in 1970. He was named president and CEO in 1982 and became chairman of the Board of Trustees on October 1, 1998.

He is a Fellow in the American College of Health Care Executives, was a founding board member of Voluntary Hospitals of America, Inc., was a founding board member/officer of the Hospital Alliance of Tennessee, and has been a member of the American Hospital Association, the American Nursing Home Association, and the South Eastern Hospital Association. He is a former member of the Governing Board of the Mid-Tennessee Eye Bank Foundation and is currently a member of the board of NationsBank of Tennessee.

Stringfield has received many honors and awards. These are just a few: the American Marketing Association Nashville Chapter named him the 1989 "Corporate Marketer of the Year"; Middle Tennessee Medical Center honored his vision and leadership by establishing a C. David Stringfield Dedicatory Plaque on the Baptist Women's Pavilion East Building in Murfreesboro; and the Nashville *Sourcebook* and *Business Nashville* have consistently named him one of the city's "one hundred most influential leaders" since such lists were first published in 1991. Stringfield himself has felt most honored by the Board of Trustees' decision to name and dedicate the C. David Stringfield Building at Baptist Hospital in December 1987.

Over the years Stringfield has had only two secretaries, first Irma Pardon and then Audrey Saleh. He has relied on both women to run his busy office efficiently, to process his correspondence, and to help him keep track of his many appointments, among other tasks. He has greatly valued them and their efforts. Stringfield said, "First impressions are always lasting! The tremendous dedication to patients, their families, and loved ones is one reason that Baptist Hospital is the preferred hospital with 97 to 98 percent of the patients saying they would return. In my thirty years everyone has had only extremely positive things to say about Irma Pardon and Audrey Saleh. They truly show Christian love and concern, and they have always worked very hard to represent Baptist Hospital as a Christian healing ministry."

The theme of Stringfield's administration has been reinvesting money in programs and services that help save patients money and help them avoid the need for hospitalization. Baptist is recognized as

Opposite page: President and CEO C. David Stringfield oversaw a period of phenomenal growth in Baptist Hospital; he became chairman of the board October 1, 1998.

"On behalf of the Metropolitan Board of Education, the citizens of Nashville and the students of our schools, I want to express our collective appreciation to you and your business for participation in our vocational cooperative education program."
—*John H. Harris Director, Metro Nashville Public Schools*

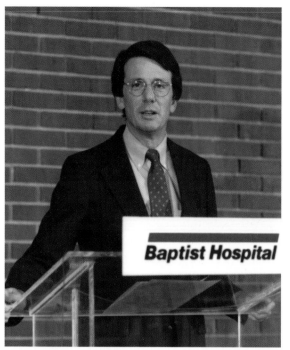

Paul Moore, executive vice president, has earned the respect of everyone from the administrative staff, medical staff, and Board of Trustees to the hospital's employees for his leadership abilities.

the low-cost, high-quality provider by patients, insurance companies, and government payers alike. And it is the industry leader in providing preventive health and wellness programs for area residents as well as business and industry.

An aggressive building program has been necessary, as Stringfield pointed out: "Health care has become so much more competitive than it used to be. If Baptist Hospital was going to survive, we had to renovate our older buildings and we had to put up new buildings and we had to put up newer facilities." But the people at the hospital cannot be overemphasized: "I think the physicians and patients want to come here because we have a magnificent group of people on the administrative staff, department heads, and grassroots employees."

On the subject of evaluating risks before undertaking a new program, Stringfield gives primary credit to the Lord. Prayer before big decisions in committee meetings and board meetings is the norm. The board is quick to act when a need is demonstrated, and the physicians offer input about new programs. They evaluate studies that have been done and visit sites, if necessary, where a program is in effect.

People who have worked with Stringfield always mention his vision. Guy Bates, immediate past chairman of the board, stated that Stringfield's "vision is just unbelievable. It's unexcelled. His capacity to accept something and review it is just unsurpassed, particularly in the administrative field of hospitals." Rev. Dr. H. Franklin Paschall, a former chairman of the board, said, "I have been a part of [the cutting edge of progress] in terms of the vision, the excitement, and the actual procurement and the achievement of those things, but give David Stringfield the credit for a creative mind and hard work. He puts in long hours. . . . He also has been fortunate in his personnel and having personnel with him who would make real contributions. The doctors are very important—if you don't have doctors, you don't have a hospital."

Paul W. Moore, current executive vice president, recalled a specific idea that increased the hospital's visibility: "David Stringfield is a marketing wizard. He had this idea that we should have a sign in the shape of a stork and give it away to the new mothers in obstetrics. Putting them out in the yards of the people in Nashville would be a good advertisement for Baptist Hospital." And it has been.

Moore earned his undergraduate degree from Rhodes College in Memphis, a doctoral degree in divinity from Vanderbilt University, and a master's degree in hospital administration from Trinity University in San Antonio. He came to Baptist Hospital in 1978 as public relations director and eventually became executive vice president in 1984. Stringfield credits Moore for his "tireless work" during the hospital's period of explosive growth. He adds, "I am so proud of Paul Moore for the great progress he has made since he began his career

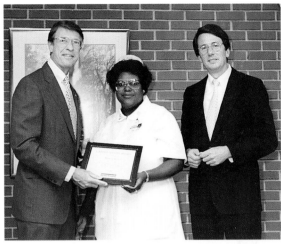

Fannie Baxter, RN, receives a prestigious Caring Hands Award from David Stringfield and Paul Moore.

at Baptist Hospital as public relations director and has justifiably been promoted to various other titles, with his current position as executive vice president. I am honored to have served with him in these many capacities for twenty years. The rank-and-file employees, the administrative staff, the medical staff, and the Board of Trustees respect him, and he deserves this respect. Paul has shown leadership not only in programs within Baptist Hospital but also in activities outside Baptist Hospital. He is the best!"

Throughout his years at the hospital, Moore has seen remarkable changes. Now he says, "There is an acceleration of changes. Things that in the past would have taken five years now must be accomplished in five months." Therefore, the challenge is "to be right the first time," but he believes the staff has a sense of optimism about embracing change and feeling comfortable with it.

"It takes a vital combination of characteristics in order to be first. You've got to have guts, because if you are wrong, then you are out there with a product that nobody wants. It's risky, but you've got to have insight. You've got to have knowledge. You've got to know what the new technology is. This is a combination of various influences from the board, from Mr. Stringfield, from medical staff," asserted Moore.

As Moore observed, the members of the Board of Trustees have been integral in the success of the hospital. Paschall addressed the duties of the board: the job is to set policy. He said, "We have to do with the planning, projecting a program and the policies pertaining" to it, but "we leave administrative matters to the administrator."

A child of the Great Depression, Paschall was concerned about the sound financial health of Baptist Hospital: "I'm financially conservative

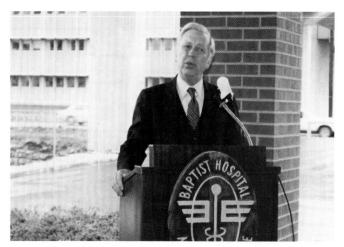

At the end of his tenure as chairman of the board, Dr. H. Franklin Paschall was honored for his efforts on behalf of the hospital by having the boardroom in the Stringfield Building named for him.

The celebration of the hospital's twenty-fifth anniversary featured people from the Billy Graham Evangelistic Association. Left to right: Tedd Smith, C. David Stringfield, Karlene Shea, George Beverly Shea, and Cliff Barrows.

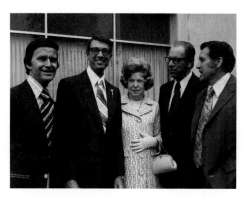

with institutions, as well as personally I'm conservative. Now we have done all this expansion and it has been phenomenal. I emphasized at every juncture, let us stay in a sound fiscal position and we have done that. We spent millions of dollars over a period of five years and our rates are below those of some hospitals and our services are superior. I'm glad that Baptist Hospital is far and away the preferred hospital for medical care in the Nashville community."

The influential industry magazine *Modern Healthcare* named Paschall Trustee of the Year in 1989 and featured him on its cover. At a special luncheon honoring Paschall, Stringfield observed, "As healthcare delivery shifted from an emphasis on long-term acute care to preventive medicine, health and fitness, and outpatient surgery, Dr. Paschall saw to it that Baptist was ahead of the pack." At the end of his term as chairman of the board in April 1989, the board room was named for Paschall.

On another occasion Stringfield paid tribute to all board members: "We are blessed enormously with having a visionary board—a board that is willing to not only keep pace with advances in medicine but to jump ahead of where the advances in medicine are going. For example, about fifteen years ago I discussed with the board what I thought was going to be the future of health care in the expansion of outpatient surgery and the board went along with that recommendation. Since that time we have expanded our outpatient surgery center several times."

Stringfield continued, "I thought—and the other administrative staff thought—there would be a greater emphasis on health, fitness, and keeping people out of the hospital by keeping them healthy, so the board was farsighted enough to endorse our recommendation to build a very fine fitness center fifteen years ago, and we are the leading hospital in the area of health promotions. I think the success of Baptist Hospital can be attributed in part to our outstanding buildings and equipment, but most of all to the personal and professional service we provide to our patients."

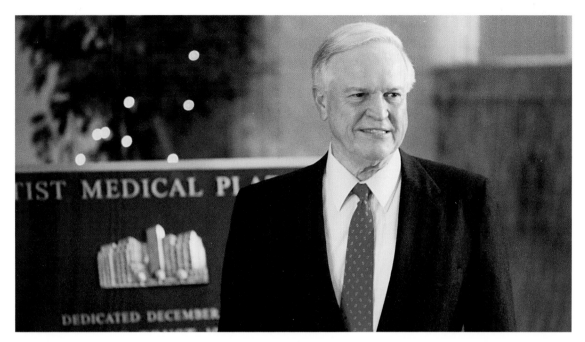

Guy Bates, who succeeded Paschall as board chairman in 1989, has been at the forefront of many changes. The Guy E. Bates Sr. Conference Center was named in his honor. He wanted to "make Baptist Hospital the flagship hospital of the South," and he recognized the need to diversify in services, particularly noting outpatient surgery. He also acknowledged other board members' roles: "We're not going to be cramped here one of these days, thanks to guys like Willie Davis and some other sharp board members who have done a wonderful job in staying ahead. We've purchased quite a bit of property and we've done it without going into debt." The hospital has room to expand if needed.

In 1991, the Tennessee Baptist Convention voted to accept a measure to change its legal relationship with Baptist Hospital. The corporation is now governed by a Board of Trustees composed of twenty-seven members which includes community members, business leaders, physicians, and religious leaders from the Middle Tennessee area. The full board meets a minimum of once a year at the annual meeting of the corporation to approve corporate matters and to approve the actions of the Executive Committee. In recent years the full board has met several times a year because of so many new and innovative programs and ideas. The board has established an Executive Committee composed of seven members of the board, which has all of the powers of the board except the reserved powers of the board

As chairman of the board from 1989 to 1998, Guy Bates offered his expertise and guidance throughout the hospital's aggressive building and acquisition programs. The Guy Bates Conference Center was dedicated in his honor on June 12, 1996.

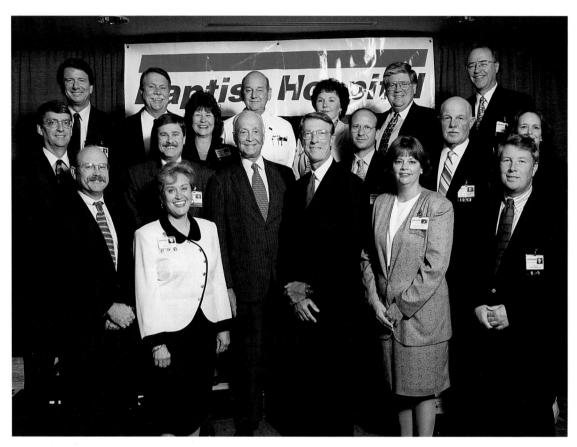

The Baptist administrative staff met with Sir John Templeton at a hospital luncheon in his honor on June 5, 1998. Left to right: Front row—Robert Rippy, Joanne Knight, C. David Stringfield, Susan Crutchfield, Lewis Lamberth Middle row—Ben Fowler, Mike Crews, Sir John Templeton, Jim Jones, Gerald Hemmer, Debby Koch Back row—Paul Moore, Art Victorine, Rachel West, Dr. Robert Hardin, Evelyn Springer, Cal MacKay, Tom Troy Not pictured—Dr. William Anderson, Jim Farris, Sue Longcore, David Purcell.

consisting of (i) authorizing distributions; (ii) approving dissolution, merger, or the sale, pledge, or transfer of all or substantially all of the corporation's assets; (iii) electing, appointing, or removing trustees or filling vacancies on the board or on any of its committees; or (iv) adopting, amending, or repealing the Charter or Bylaws of the corporation. The Executive Committee serves as the governing body for the corporation and as such performs all duties of the planning committee, finance and audit committee, and other committees as needed. (Board members are listed in the appendixes.)

The hospital also receives advice from the Baptist Health Care System Board, whose members are recommended by the Tennessee Baptist Convention. (Board members are listed in the appendixes.)

Baptist Hospital is fortunate to have a Corporate Board of community leaders. It consists of thirty-nine of the top CEOs in the community, representing the largest and most influential companies. These leaders meet quarterly with hospital administrators to learn about healthcare advancements and challenges, and to provide their unique perspective from corporate America to Baptist Hospital decision makers. (Current members are listed in the appendixes.)

Over the years, the administrators and the board have seen to it that the hospital sought accreditation. In 1953, Mid-State Baptist Hospital was fully approved by the American College of Surgeons, by the American Medical Association—Council on Medical Education for the training of interns and residents, and by the Tennessee Board of Nursing to operate an accredited school of nursing. The hospital was a member of the American Hospital Association, American Protestant Hospital Association, and Tennessee Hospital Association.

Baptist received a score of 97 percent on its most recent Joint Commission on the Accreditation of Healthcare Organizations survey in 1996—the highest in the region and among the highest in the country.

The costs in general to operate the hospital have grown exponentially, and the joint efforts of the administrative staff, the board, and the medical staff have been effective in keeping services cost-effective, yet high quality. It is hard to believe that rates in 1947 at Protestant Hospital were from $5.50 to $12 per day for a bed. The average daily cost of operating Baptist Hospital in 1955 was about $5,000; in 1965, almost $16,000; in 1975, more than $65,000; in 1985, more than $196,000; and in 1997, more than $717,000.

A major contributing factor to the dramatic rise in operating costs was the advancement in medical technology. "The volume of surgical and medical supplies consumed by the hospital multiplied many times over," according to Glen Sesler, a longtime Baptist Hospital employee who was vice president of purchasing at the time of his retirement. "The explosion of new technology placed new challenges on our inventory and distribution systems, but we accommodated. I've always been proud that Baptist provided the very latest, most advanced medical equipment and supplies for our physicians and nurses."

Of course the gross revenues of the hospital have grown too: in 1948, $479,153; in 1955, $1,954,389; in 1965, $7,409,801; in 1985, $106,323,598; and in 1995, $399,662,308.

The present workforce of more than 2,800 people and more than 1,000 physicians makes

"After my operation I had the kindest nurse waiting on me every day until 3 o'clock. . . . Her name was Mrs. Wilma Gooch."
—Mrs. F. L. Heery

Left to right:
Guy Bates, Virgil Moore Jr., and Rev. Virgil Peters at the ground breaking for the Mid State Garage.

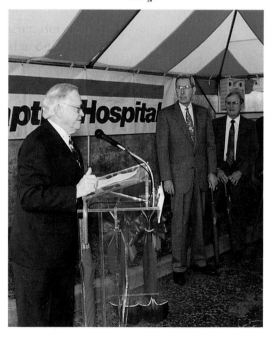

"I suffered a very tragic accident. I hurt my leg very badly when my riding lawn mower turned over on me. I asked the ambulance personnel to take me to Baptist Hospital. I was in surgery that night to save my leg. Your life changes dramatically when you have eight surgeries in twelve days. I spent thirty days in the orthopedic unit, twenty-six of those flat on my back. . . . The Baptist doctors and nurses not only saved my leg, they helped me through this most traumatic time."

—*Rick Regen*

Baptist Hospital the tenth largest employer in Nashville. Rachel West, assistant vice president of Human Resources, said that a competitive salary and benefit package is important to recruiting employees. However, her job is made easier because Baptist has a "reputation for being the most caring hospital." West has seen "unbelievable growth in new programs and services at Baptist Hospital for patients. That applies equally to programs to satisfy employees." An example is Baptist Hospital Child Care, which has been in existence about ten years. Baptist was the first client of Corporate Family Solutions and the first hospital in the area to open its own child care center.

Another way that Baptist recognizes the vital work of its employees is through the Caring Hands Award. The award goes to members of the Baptist family whose actions demonstrate that they care about patients, patients' families, fellow employees, and the caring mission of Baptist Hospital in an exceptional manner. Three hundred employees have received the award since it began in 1988. Employees vote on who should get the award. The name Caring Hands came from a mission hospital in South America that stood out above all other mission hospitals in meeting needs of the community and patients. Local people would walk for days, often carrying a sick person, to get to the mission hospital for aid, and some would pass by other hospitals. They explained why they would do that: "At this hospital, the hands are different." Baptist Hospital is achieving the same thing.

For its twenty-fifth anniversary, the hospital chose the theme: Serving the Brotherhood of Man for 25 Years. In attendance on April 26, 1973, were Mayor Beverly Briley, Governor Winfield Dunn, Congressman Dick Fulton, Senators Howard Baker and Bill Brock, and representatives of the Tennessee Baptist Convention and the Southern Baptist Convention. The celebration featured Cliff Barrows, George Beverly Shea, and Tedd Smith of the Billy Graham Evangelistic Association.

To celebrate 80 Years of Caring, Baptist Hospital has held free health screenings for the community throughout 1998: January—iron screening (hemachromatosis); February—heart; March—ovarian cancer, prenatal vitamin campaign, and Diabetes Alert Day; April—Childbirth Fair; May—skin cancer and athletic screenings; June—osteoporosis; July—colorectal; August—heart; September—prostate cancer; October—breast cancer; November—diabetes; and December—stress.

National leaders and an internationally distributed magazine have paid tribute to Baptist Hospital for its accomplishments. During a visit to Baptist in 1992, then Secretary of Health and Human Services Louis Sullivan, M.D., said that Baptist's "commitment to a healthy nation is unparalleled. Your dedication and continued education and preventive health programming will help to bring us one step closer to improving the quality of life for all Americans."

An October 1993 article in *The Economist* cited Nashville's health-care industry as an example of the problems and solutions faced in American health care and pointed to Baptist Hospital as "one hospital in the city positioned for success."

Former President George Bush joined hospital executives in 1994 to unveil a new independent survey that showed Baptist with the highest in-hospital survival rates and the lowest hospital charges for two critical heart procedures—coronary artery bypass and heart valve replacement surgery. The research findings were outlined in the "Performance Report on Cardiovascular Procedures" compiled by Healthcare Data Source of Englewood, Colorado, a national healthcare data research firm.

In addition, internal surveys of patients report that 98 percent who come to Baptist Hospital say they would return to Baptist if they had to be rehospitalized. Stringfield says, "In every marketing survey that is taken of Baptist Hospital, we are the leading hospital with the exception of one category. Vanderbilt is perceived to have the latest equipment by the public and I think rightfully so because it is a teaching/research hospital. But for us to lead all the other hospitals—not by a little bit but sometimes four to one, and in some cases ten to one—in these marketing surveys, as having the friendliest staff, most caring nursing staff, best food, cleanest hospital—right on down the road to every marketing category—that's the reason for Baptist's successes."

Baptist Hospital and its affiliate in Smithville, Baptist DeKalb Hospital, were named to the 1995 list of "100 Top Hospitals: Benchmarks for Success." The study of nearly 3,500 acute-care hospitals nationwide is annually performed and compiled by HCIA, Inc., and Mercer Health Provider Consulting. The purpose of the study is to "identify a set of benchmarks for the hospital industry that represent a balance of high quality care, efficient delivery and superior financial performance. Specific criteria included each facility's levels of outpatient activity, mortality and morbidity ratios, length of stay, profitability and expenses per discharge."

In 1996, Baptist Hospital was named one of the nation's quality healthcare leaders, the only Middle Tennessee facility recognized and only one of five in the state. Survey results by the National Research

"My doctor insisted that I go to Baptist for further tests. I'm in my mid-forties and I never really thought much about heart trouble. And then one day, chest pains came. By-pass surgery from a clogged artery may have saved my life. The Heart Center rehab nurses have been my guardian angels, They have inspired me to get back to a full and active life without fear. Thanks Baptist for the new lease on life!"
—Paul Scheil

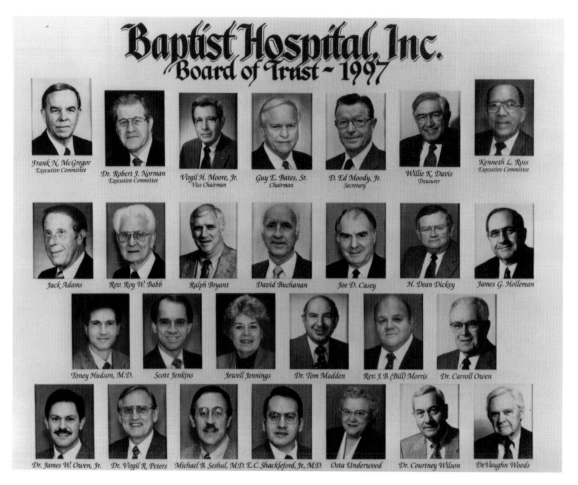

Baptist Hospital, Inc.
Board of Trust ~ 1997

Frank N. McGregor
Executive Committee

Dr. Robert J. Norman
Executive Committee

Virgil H. Moore, Jr.
Vice Chairman

Guy E. Bates, Sr.
Chairman

D. Ed Moody, Jr.
Secretary

Willie K. Davis
Treasurer

Kenneth L. Ross
Executive Committee

Jack Adams

Rev. Roy W. Babb

Ralph Bryant

David Buchanan

Joe D. Casey

H. Dean Dickey

James G. Holleman

Toney Hudson, M.D.

Scott Jenkins

Jewell Jennings

Dr. Tom Madden

Rev. J. B (Bill) Morris

Dr. Carroll Owen

Dr. James W. Owen, Jr.

Dr. Virgil R. Peters

Michael B. Seshul, M.D.

E.C. Shackleford, Jr., M.D.

Osta Underwood

Dr. Courtney Wilson

DeVaughn Woods

Much of Baptist Hospital's success can be attributed to the cooperative attitudes of board members, administrative staff, and medical staff. These board members have fostered that spirit of cooperation. These are the men and women who served on the board during the hospitals ten year, $300 million building and expansion program.

Corporation were announced in *Modern Healthcare*. The next year, 1997, Baptist was again honored in this public opinion poll. The primary healthcare decision maker within each household polled named the hospital he or she would choose first for all household healthcare needs. Overall preference measures opinions specific to hospitals with the best physicians/nurses, image/reputation, quality, community health programs, and most personalized care. Stringfield noted, "Our mission has always been to provide the community with high-quality, compassionate health care, delivered in the most cost-effective manner possible. This honor is especially gratifying to us because it is based on public preferences among area hospitals." The hospital's administrators and board have worked hard to meet this mission and will continue to meet it in the future.

Chapter 6

MEDICAL TEAMS AND TECHNOLOGICAL ADVANCES

Nashville benefits from a quality of medical practice higher than for most places of its size in the United States. And that goes beyond competence of the physicians in their respective fields to their ethical nature.
— *John M. Tudor, M.D.*

"FIVE YEARS AGO THIS HOSPITAL HAD ONE INTERN and no residents. Today we count with pride an ever-growing house staff that on the first of this July will number twenty full-time graduate doctors. The hospital now has a full-time specialist in Pathology in charge of the laboratories; a full-time doctor anesthetist with five well-trained nurse anesthetists; a School of Nursing with a large staff of well-trained teachers and supervisors. And so it has been with each department: a constant growth in order to render a better service." These comments, which appeared in a booklet for the 1953 dedication of the South Building, spelled out many improvements that occurred in the five years following the hospital's change in ownership.

World War II had wide-ranging effects on the arena of medical practice, and hospitals needed to have several departments. Protestant

Hospital—and then Mid-State Baptist Hospital in its early years—was "by and for general practice physicians," according to John M. Tudor, M.D., who became associated with Mid-State Baptist Hospital in 1950. There had been only four or five specialties before the war, but World War II was "paramount in fostering the specialty practice of medicine" and organized medicine had to respond to the change.

Dr. Tudor regarded Gene Kidd as an administrator "who recognized the importance of having a solidly based, competent medical staff," and he worked to provide that for Baptist. He made "an old hospital attractive to specialists."

Having specialty training in urology, Dr. Tudor joined an existing staff led by Dr. Oscar Carter and Dr. Charles Haines. By 1953, the twelve services at Baptist included internal medicine, radiology, general practice, otolaryngology, pathology, orthopaedics, dentistry, urology, anesthesiology, surgery, obstetrics, and pediatrics. The twelve services with chiefs in 1977 were anesthesiology, family practice, internal medicine, medical imaging, obstetrics/gynecology, ophthalmology, orthopaedics, otolaryngology, pathology, pediatrics, surgery, and urology. A year later emergency medicine was added as a service, then psychiatry in 1989, and plastic surgery and neuroscience in 1992.

Oscar Carter, M.D., who was a noted urologist for fifty years at the hospital, retired with a party in his honor.
Left to right:
C. David Stringfield,
Dr. Mike Spalding,
Dr. Tom Nesbitt Sr.,
Dr. Oscar Carter, Dr. John Tudor,
Paul W. Moore,
Dr. Tom Nesbitt Jr.,
Dr. Robert McClellan.

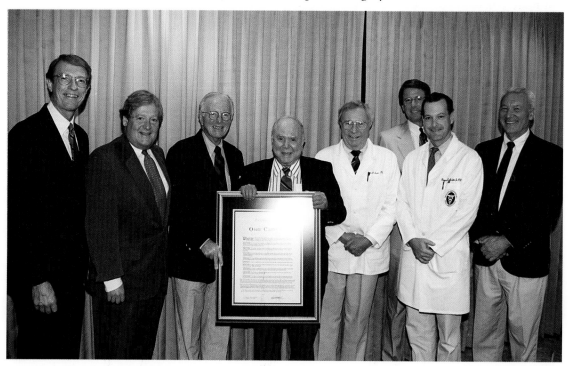

The chief of medical staff held an unpaid position. He saw to it that physicians were properly credentialed; he did peer reviews, ensured quality of care, and dealt with the rare disciplinary issues relating to the medical staff. In essence, the chief of staff was the physician responsible to the Board of Trustees and the public. Carrying out his duties required a tremendous commitment of time and effort.

A 1955 brochure about Mid-State Baptist Hospital called it a general, short-term hospital. There were no facilities for mental, contagious, or chronic/convalescent patients. Baptist was accredited by the Joint Commission Accreditation of Hospitals.

Training was fairly diverse for a hospital of its size. In 1956 there were rotating internships and residencies in obstetrics/gynecology, internal medicine, pediatrics, surgery, and pathology. The School of Oxygen Therapy offered two-year on-the-job training to inhalation therapists. Few hospitals had an Inhalation Therapy Department then. There was a School of X-Ray Technology, and Edgar Byrd, a medical technologist, founded Baptist Medical School of Technology in that year. About 150 students completed the twelve-month course before the Baptist Medical School of Technology closed in the 1980s.

In the 1950s, 1960s, and early 1970s, Nashville hospitals probably had more patients from outside Middle Tennessee than they do now because fewer areas had specialists. People would come from Georgia, Alabama, and Mississippi. Nashville and Memphis were the centers for higher levels of medical care. Dr. Tudor recalled that in his specialty of urology in the 1940s and 1950s, only eight or ten top-notch training programs existed in the United States.

Then a reversal in the trend developed as training of specialists proliferated in the late 1970s and early 1980s. There were better and more training programs. Medical centers were saturated with specialists.

In the Vietnam War era some physicians were recalled following the reinstitution of the physician draft. Some were gone two or three years and then came back to Baptist. (No physicians from Baptist who had been in World War II were recalled to the Korean War.) John Wright, M.D., was one who was recalled and was decorated for his work in Vietnam. His service to Baptist also deserves commendation. During his many years of tenure as chief of surgery, Dr. Wright judiciously monitored the service.

In Dr. Tudor's experience, Baptist "has been in the forefront of urology, orthopaedics, and neuro-otology." To him, the "giants" at the hospital have been Dr. Oscar Carter in urology, Dr. Ben Fowler in orthopaedics, Dr. Michael E. Glasscock III in neuro-otology, and Dr.

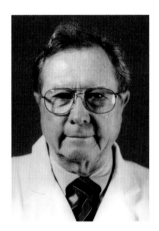

The first Medical Affairs Director of the hospital was John M. Tudor, M.D.

Arthur Bond in neurosurgery. Dr. Carter set a record on the number of transurethral resections, and in addition to being a pioneer in total hip replacement surgery and a highly skilled surgeon of the hand, Dr. Fowler was the founder and director of the Rehabilitation Center. "Dr. Fowler was deeply respected for his medical staff vision and often consulted by administration, nursing service, and Board of Trustees on many matters. Even following his retirement from medical practice, he was contacted frequently to get his thoughts on the future of medicine and the role that Baptist Hospital should take," according to David Stringfield.

That being said, Dr. Tudor maintains that Baptist has always had a full complement of excellent physicians on the medical staff. Russell Birmingham, M.D., was one who served in many capacities over the years: chief of obstetrics/gynecological service, chief of staff, president of the medical staff, and a member of the Executive Committee of the Board of Trustees. Elkin Rippy, M.D., was a leader of the medical staff, often referred to as the "mayor of the medical staff" as he presided over and directed discussions in the doctors' lounge. He has been

The operating room is prepared for surgery, pre-1980.

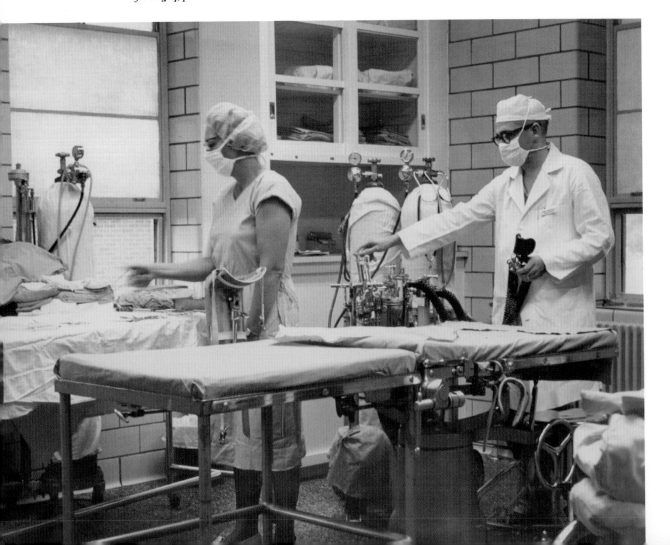

known for his common sense and sense of humor as much as for his efforts in composing a great deal of the bylaws of the medical staff. Stringfield commented, "Dr. Rippy had a very colorful and interesting medical practice, for he practiced during the time that physicians made house calls and provided a great deal of charity care. He was a fine general surgeon with a variety of interests, such as a songwriter and an author of three humorous books. He also assisted in architectural designs of buildings."

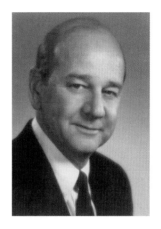

A longtime cardiac surgeon at Baptist, Robert A. Hardin, M.D., is the current Medical Affairs Director.

Presently, Baptist Hospital has an educational affiliation with Vanderbilt that goes back to the late 1960s and early 1970s. Vanderbilt residents in urology, obstetrics, and plastic surgery rotate through Baptist as part of their training.

By the mid-1980s, the need for a full-time Medical Affairs Director became apparent because of changes in health care and more bureaucracy demanding compliance. The daily implementation problems eased with the director's appointment. The chief of staff, a practicing physician, remained a primary person involved in disciplinary issues.

Dr. Tudor assumed the Medical Affairs Director position in 1985 and left it in 1997 to return to private practice. The director is responsible for meeting the needs of the medical staff and providing logistical support for the chief of staff. In effect, he is the facilitator for the chiefs of services and the chief of staff. The bylaws stipulate a chief of staff, chiefs of services, and a Performance Improvement Committee, among other committees. Each department credentials its own members; Medical Staff Services keep all records straight and up to date.

Robert A. Hardin, M.D., became Medical Affairs Director after Dr. Tudor. He was Associate Medical Director for three years before that. He has seen four parts to the job: (1) verifying that physicians have proper credentials; (2) assuring quality, called performance improvement at Baptist, which includes monitoring mortality, infection, and return to surgery rates; (3) serving as liaison between medical staff and administration; and (4) resolving problems brought by patients in regard to a physician's care. Compared to earlier years, the regulations in regard to certification of physicians have become stricter, and meeting those requirements has become more time-consuming for all involved.

Dr. Hardin has been at Baptist for thirty-four years. A cardiac surgeon, he graduated from Vanderbilt Medical School in 1956, did his surgical residency at Indiana University Medical Center after serving in the U.S. Army Medical Corps, then came to Baptist. He has always considered Baptist a "broad-based" care hospital. Diversity is a strength

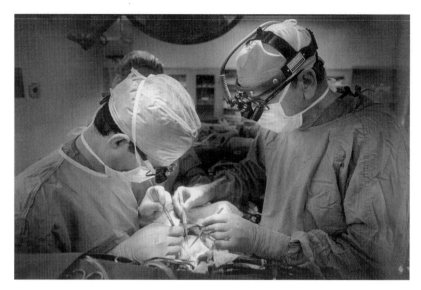

Dr. Kenneth Laws, left, and Dr. Robert Hardin, right, perform cardiac surgery.

that brings balance to the hospital so that not all care is in one field. For example, although open-heart surgery was performed at Baptist in 1971, right after Saint Thomas's first open-heart surgeries, Baptist chose not to become a one-specialty hospital.

Six operating rooms were available in Dr. Hardin's early years at Baptist. Now there are seventeen operating rooms in the main surgical area of the hospital, a separate laser suite with six operating rooms, an Outpatient Surgery Center with fourteen operating rooms, and another free-standing Outpatient Surgery Center with four more operating rooms.

From an administrator's point of view, David Stringfield stressed that a primary reason for Baptist hospital's success is attributed to the fact that it is a doctors' hospital: "We ask doctors to give us input as to what they think we can do to make Baptist a better hospital. We have planning sessions with them on a periodic basis. We involve not just a certain group of doctors, but we involve ourselves with different groups of doctors each time we have a planning session. The members of the medical staff have enormous impact in terms of recommending what they think the future of health care should hold and how they think we should deal with it. This year, 1998, we have 1,088 doctors on our medical staff." (The number was slightly more than 300 in 1955, about 400 in the late 1960s and early 1970s, and more than 550 in 1980.)

Stringfield recognized that "the ultimate delivery of health care is in the hands of the physicians who practice medicine at Baptist, and we have worked diligently to help members of the medical staff to better serve their patients. This includes constructing medical office buildings and parking facilities near the hospital, installing special equipment which the physicians need to keep pace with advancing technology, and constantly listening and responding to their suggestions about improving care."

He added, "We try to run the type of hospital that will attract the most qualified and respected physicians in the area to practice here, and to offer such superior facilities and services that Baptist will be their hospital of choice. Our goal is to be the best hospital in Middle Tennessee with outstanding physicians." In fact, Baptist Hospital is a small city with thousands of patients, outpatients, employees, physicians, and visitors on hand each day.

The physicians who formed Baptist Healthcare Group (BHG), with an emphasis on primary care, in the early 1990s had previously belonged to another group at another hospital. According to J. Michael Bolds, M.D., they made the move to Baptist so that they could have the "opportunity to grow." And they have been successful in accomplishing their goal because the original group of eleven has grown to twenty-one physicians and one nurse practitioner in the offices on the Baptist Hospital campus. Dr. Bolds believes that Baptist is a "hospital that has won the hearts of the residents of Davidson County." In this "turbulent time" in the practice of medicine, he says that Baptist is a "durable institution that has weathered many changes in health care and is adaptable to meeting the new realities of the healthcare world." From the administrative staff to the first-class physicians, Dr. Bolds sees that Baptist is "committed to a very high quality of patient care."

One of the physicians who worked at Baptist for many years (1971–97) and thought of it as a doctors' hospital was Michael E. Glasscock III, a neuro-otologist. His patients came from Middle Tennessee and the surrounding area as well as from all over the world: Israel, Sri Lanka, Canada, South America, and South Africa. He was the largest single admitter in the 1970s and 1980s. He felt that both Gene Kidd and David Stringfield saw to it that Baptist was a well-run hospital and they got what physicians needed in a timely manner.

Like Dr. Tudor, Dr. Glasscock noted the hospital's emphasis on urology, neurology, and orthopaedics. Early in his career, Dr. Glasscock set out to build a specially trained team of the same people in the same operating room, and he had that for almost twenty years. Now teams are common, such as the open-heart team, the ENT team, and the neurosurgery team.

"I want to commend your staff that works in the Emergency Room at night. We had a group of students in Nashville, and one of them, a 16-year-old from Denmark, had to be treated. . . . All of you restored our faith in human kindness and medical professionalism."

—Bill Hampton
Principal, Obion County
High School

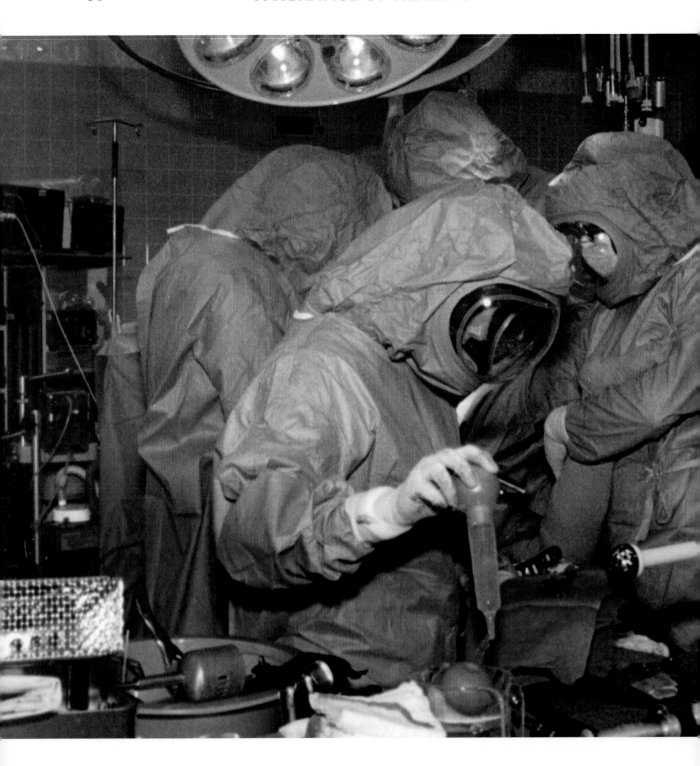

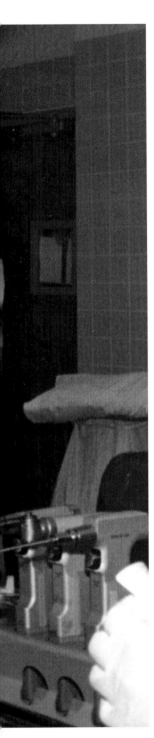

A big problem to him was that "insurance companies are dictating medicine." He "never let insurance companies dictate what procedure was needed or the length of stay." His priorities were the patient and a good outcome. After all, as he said, "Nobody can practice medicine but doctors."

Dr. Tudor remarked that "doctors are losing their grip on how to deliver health care." He has seen big changes in how things have happened, yet "managed care in the long run is not going to save a lot of money." To some degree patient care may revert to the old patient-physician relationship, but he thinks there will be less fee-for-service. More younger physicians are willing to be salaried employees of hospitals, and fewer physicians are creating their own small businesses. For-profit hospitals might have provided some better medicine to some smaller communities; nevertheless, he believed that the "entrepreneurs in health care have had an overall negative effect."

Charles E. Mayes, M.D., is a cardiologist who performed the first angioplasty at Baptist Hospital in 1980. He had joined the practice of Constantine Potanin, M.D., in 1976. To him, these are the "best of times" because of the medical and technological advances that improve the quality of care for patients. He believes that "medicine is a calling," and he continues to find it gratifying to practice medicine at Baptist Hospital. However, these are the "worst of times" because of the overwhelming number of rules and regulations associated with the bureaucracy of state and local governments and insurance companies.

In Dr. Hardin's opinion, bureaucracy is becoming even more of a problem and the government is becoming even more intrusive and making more regulations. A possible and undesirable outcome is that the government intrusion may drive some physicians out of practice because they are tired of the hassles of "getting permission from accountants to practice medicine." More of the "sharp edge of consumers is backing up against government."

This photo from the early 1970s illustrates the special suits designed to protect the sterile environment during joint replacement surgery. Similar suits are still in use today.

T. Guv Pennington, M.D., has come from a long line of physicians. Both parents practiced at Protestant Hospital, and his brother is also a physician. Dr. Guv Pennington started practicing at Baptist in 1957, with a specialty in internal medicine; he later added a subspecialty in allergies. In those early days he had patients at all the hospitals in town; in addition, he made house calls and taught at General Hospital and Vanderbilt. Now he teaches in the University of Tennessee-Baptist Hospital Internal Medicine Residency Program. Gradually, he and the other doctors in Nashville allied with one hospital, and he chose Baptist. "In addition to serving in many capacities on the medical staff, Dr. Pennington often responded to requests for his insights from the administration and Board of Trustees. His guidance in establishing the residency program in primary care associated with the University of Tennessee was phenomenal, and his leadership will be appreciated by future generations," said Stringfield.

As a member of Heritage Medical Associates, Dr. Pennington and his colleagues counted the number of insurance companies with which they do business—twenty-eight—and each one has different payment procedures, rates, rules, and regulations. He has seen patients reacting negatively to such policies as managed care dictating that each patient is allotted only ten to twelve minutes. "That is no way to have to practice medicine; something is going to have to change," he said. He summed up his philosophy about being a doctor: "I've done a lot of teaching over the years. Students will come up to me and say, 'Would you advise a young person to go into medicine?' I answer, 'It depends on your priorities. If you're in it for money or ego, you're in it for the wrong reasons. But if you love to take care of patients, you'll always make money and you'll always enjoy it.'"

Since 1969, H. Newt Lovvorn Jr., M.D., has practiced at Baptist Hospital as an obstetrician/gynecologist. He says, "The pendulum is swinging too far in cutting payments to physicians. The pendulum will swing back." Setting up a single-physician practice is cost-prohibitive to younger physicians just starting out, and older ones have found advantages in forming groups. Dr. Lovvorn has joined with a few other doctors—and they have plans to enlarge the group even more—in order to make the practice more efficient. He said that being able to "get various heads together on a difficult case" benefits the patients. Over the years, he has done fertility work, obstetrical work, and now pelvic support surgery. He has been able to go through life stages with his patients—from childbearing years to menopause—and has enjoyed being at Baptist, a "great hospital."

Edmond F. Tipton, M.D., has made a unique response to some of the problems associated with health care. He has assumed a teaching position as an associate professor at Belmont University's Massey Graduate School of Business in the area of healthcare management. As a physician with years of clinical experience, he hopes to have a positive effect on what the students learn, "to teach them the ethical, emotional aspects in regard to decisions" about health care. He wants to "marry the two—professional ethics and business rules—and be successful in not violating either one." He said, "It is easy for people to say, 'Health care is inefficient.'" But the public needs to participate in all facets of the discussion to figure out a better system. Having practiced in pulmonology and internal medicine with expertise in respiratory therapy since 1979 at Baptist Hospital, he saw improvements in both technology and pharmacology. Over the years the physical plant at Baptist improved greatly and its medical staff just got better and better.

More procedures done on an outpatient basis, more very sick patients who will require expanded intensive care units, and demanding baby boomers who want to be a part of what is happening in their health care are only some of the forces facing the hospital in the future. More knowledge, more training, and more technological advances are also in the hospital's future.

For example, the Center for Medical Education has a graduate medical education program affiliated with the University of Tennessee College of Medicine, focusing on primary care practi-

The PET scanner is an important diagnostic tool for physicians to use in cardiac care.

tioners. Until this program came into place, Baptist Hospital was considered a surgeons' hospital. Stringfield commented, "I saw Baptist Hospital as primarily a surgery-oriented hospital, and with managed care and the 'gatekeeper' approach, I felt it necessary to strengthen the internal medicine and primary care programs. With the guidance initially of T. Guy Pennington and other primary care physicians, a residency program in primary care was

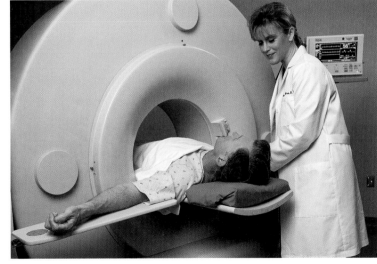

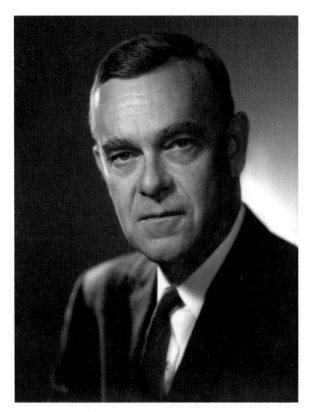

Dr. Benjamin Fowler was a pioneer in total joint replacement at Baptist Hospital where he performed the first total hip replacement in the region.

established with the University of Tennessee College of Medicine. The hospital was quite fortunate to have Paul McNabb, M.D., assume the directorship of the program, and since its inception, I have heard only positive comments about the program. This speaks well for the outstanding faculty and residents that were recruited." The center holds about 20 major conferences, featuring dermatology, orthopaedics, obstetrics/gynecology, or primary care, and almost 350 smaller conferences per year with approximately 3,500 attendees in all.

Orthopaedics has been a specialty in the Regen family for two generations. Eugene M. Regen Jr., M.D., practiced with his father for about twenty years, and Dr. Regen Jr. and Ben Fowler, M.D., traveled to Europe at various times to learn about hip replacement technology from early pioneers in the field and bring it back to Baptist Hospital. Dr. Regen Jr. designed one or two medical instruments used in the technology's infancy, and so did Dr. Fowler. He predicts a bright future for joint replacement as better and better methods and materials are perfected, and he believes the management of complicated fractures is on the verge of significant breakthroughs.

Ronald E. Overfield, M.D., a specialist in medical imaging, believes that the contributions of the computer cannot be overemphasized. In his field one can hardly keep up with the rapid developments, and in the years since he began his practice in 1969, the computer has "brought both space requirements and many prices down" as the equipment size has decreased and the complexity has increased. To him, "technology makes it easier to provide good patient care."

The role of Silicon Valley is yet to be determined in offering technological breakthroughs in medicine, but Dr. Hardin predicted a major impact. Perhaps more high-tech machines will change methods of diagnosis—a patient dials in, a physician looks at her over a monitor, and she does not go in to his office unless a procedure is indicated. Similar technology is already in place. Equipment that just a few years ago was reality only on *Star Trek* and in science fiction books is now medical reality. Baptist has a list of "firsts" in technology and treatments of which it can be proud:

1962—Medical Intensive Care Unit with twelve beds, first of its kind in the area.

1964—four-bed cardiac unit, first of its kind in the Mid-South.

1969—a $60,000 radioactive isotope unit acquired.

1971—first open-heart surgery at Baptist Hospital; first total hip replacement.

1973—first hospital in the central South to implant a nuclear-powered cardiac pacemaker, the fourth U.S. license.

1974—area's first hospital to install a new diagnostic tool, the Xerox 125 System for Xeroradiography, to help in the fight against cancer. The system produced dry pictures on paper without a darkroom to help radiologists detect breast tumors and hairline fractures. It took ninety seconds to produce the pictures.

1975—one-hundred-bed Progressive Care Center opened.

1976–77—CAT scanner and ultrasound equipment purchased; opening of the hemodialysis unit.

1985—first lithotripter in the area, one of only eleven U.S. facilities with a federally approved lithotripter (Greek for "stone crusher"). By the winter of 1986, 170 patients had been treated and 103 more scheduled for the Dornier Lithotripter. Actual treatment uses shock waves to crush kidney stones. First free-standing Outpatient Surgery Center in the region opened in Plaza I.

1986—Magnetic Resonance Imaging (MRI) undertaken.

1990—nation's first Laparoscopy and Laser Center, with six operating rooms solely for these procedures.

1995—nation's first specially constructed, self-contained Early Morning Admission Unit.

1996—PET (Positron Emission Tomography) scanner for cardiac imaging. Its goal is to lower risk and even reverse heart disease through a noninvasive technology.

1997—the first hospital in Tennessee to earn accreditation from the American College of Radiology for its stereotactic breast biopsy programs through the Women's Pavilion Health Center. The process, compared to traditional biopsies, is less expensive, leaves minimal scarring, and is virtually painless. It is an outpatient procedure with local anesthesia.

1997—Chest Pain Observation Unit of Emergency Pavilion, first of its kind in Middle Tennessee. The eight-bed unit allows patients experiencing signs of heart attack to have tests without being admitted to the hospital.

"I went in for a routine physical, and my physician referred me to the Baptist Cardiac Center, the Heart Center, and it was there that the ultimate finding of my problem took place. Baptist Hospital means quality care and professionals looking at you as an individual."

—Ben Tyler

Technology has had such a positive impact on our lives in many ways that we sometimes forget how much has been achieved in such a short time. Physicians continue to do a better job of getting patients well with newer, more powerful drugs and equipment. Modern science and more skilled personnel really have produced modern miracles. No one alive in the 1950s can forget the polio epidemic that killed many children and paralyzed others, leaving them to use wheelchairs, braces, or iron lungs. The worst year—1952—saw 58,000 cases nationwide. Then the 1955 Salk vaccine was used in shots in a dramatic public health effort, and in 1961, the sugar cubes with Sabin vaccine were handed out to children. In 1961, babies born in the hospital had a three times better chance of survival than they did just one generation before that.

Miss Daisy, a robot that takes specimens back and forth from the processing area to specialized divisions, made her debut in the Baptist Laboratory in December 1997. The walking and talking robot allows the staff to concentrate on other tasks, and she does her job for less than $6 per hour.

Members of the medical staff at Baptist are always looking for and evaluating the most up-to-date ways to help their patients. They attend conferences, do on-site visits to see firsthand a new procedure or device, read medical journals, and talk to their colleagues across the nation and around the world. Their care and compassion complement their medical expertise so that Baptist Hospital can continue to provide excellent services to the people of the community.

Chapter 7

BUILDING AND ACQUISITION PROGRAMS

When the present expansion program is completed, the hospital will stabilize at 550 beds and 75 bassinets.
—*Hospital brochure, 1961*

THE COPYWRITER OF THAT 1961 BROCHURE COULD have had no idea that the hospital's expansion program had a long way to go! What seemed to be needed then pales in comparison to the building program set forth only twenty years later. In 1948, the hospital had 210 beds and 18 bassinets. The numbers increased to 300 beds and 55 bassinets by 1959, and to 600 beds and 64 bassinets by the end of 1973. In 1998, Baptist Hospital is licensed for 759 beds. Admissions rose over the years from 6,109 inpatients in 1951 to 28,497 inpatients and 268,456 outpatient registrations (this number includes surgical procedures as well as diagnostic and therapeutic services) in 1997. To care for all the patients, more buildings and facilities were required.

The campus in 1948 consisted primarily of the East and West Buildings with four stories each and partial basements. By 1953, the dedication of the six-story South Building added 140 beds and 18 bassinets at a cost of $1.5 million. Included were a chapel, a modern dietary department, with an air-conditioned cafeteria open to visitors, a new X-ray department, a new clinical laboratory, a new obstetrics department and nursery, which were air-conditioned, and a 28–bed pediatric unit in addition to two complete floors for medical and surgical adult patients—all air-conditioned.

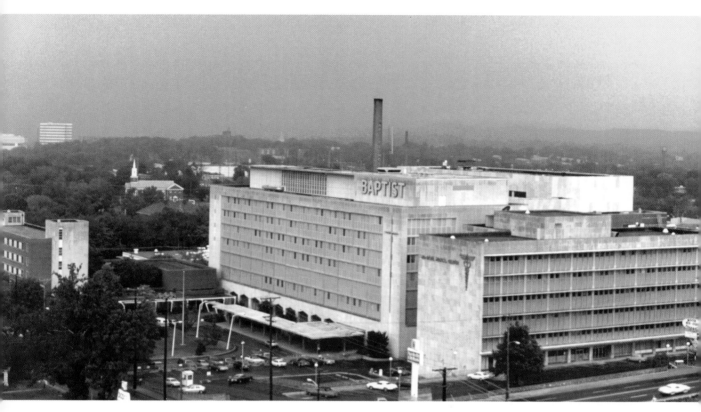

Baptist Hospital campus,
before extensive growth.

In the dedication program, Jack C. Massey, chairman of the Board of Trustees, noted that "our Baptist Hospital is staffed with the finest trained physicians in the world, a capable and proven hospital administrator, and a corps of assistants, nurses and attendants, technicians and dietitians. The skill of our physicians and surgeons is unsurpassed. We shall continue to count on those in positions of responsibility to ever strive to better every phase of service and continue to grow as the needs of our community require." The building was considered a milestone of progress, the result of much planning, praying, and working.

Other structures completed in the 1950s include the following: 1954, Intern Residences; 1955, a new West Building for the School of Nursing; and 1957, Medical Arts Auditorium. Also in 1957, thanks to a Ford Foundation grant of $138,500, the seventy-bed, self-contained wing called the Ford Annex was finished. A particularly notable achievement by 1957 was that 75 percent of the hospital was air-conditioned with central and window units, no small comfort to patients in the South in the summertime. A free-standing state-of-the-art laundry was completed in 1959.

More ambitious projects filled the 1960s. In 1960, the Mid-State Baptist Medical Center was built adjacent to the south patient wing. Local physicians had office space connected to the hospital, and that trend has become more popular over time. The Neonatal Intensive Special Care Nursery opened in 1961; a twelve-bed Medical Intensive Care Unit opened in 1962; a new $400,000 Emergency Pavilion opened in 1963; and the first Coronary Care Unit in Nashville opened at Baptist in 1964. In 1967, the old West Building was demolished to make way for the Central Building. The dedication of the Central Building in 1968 coincided with the twentieth anniversary of the hospital's new relationship with the Tennessee Baptist Convention; the hospital campus then covered two square blocks.

The eight-story, $8 million Central Building contained seventeen operating rooms in the Operating Pavilion adjoined by the Surgical Intensive Care Unit and a twenty-five-bed Recovery Unit. It also had the laboratory, radiology, dietary facilities (a kitchen, dining room space for three hundred, a snack shop, private dining rooms for physicians, Central Services, and Medical Imaging), and space for the pharmacy and other departments such as data processing. The Department of Religion occupied a suite of offices, a pastor's study, a family room, and a new chapel. This addition made Baptist the largest hospital in Middle Tennessee with 625 beds and 80 bassinets.

The final major improvement of the decade was made in 1969—a twenty-two-bed Coronary Care Unit. And 1970 saw the opening of a Cardiopulmonary Lab.

Baptist Hospital purchased five structures of the old Saint Thomas Hospital on Hayes Street for $1.5 million on August 15, 1975. Baptist Board of Trustees member Russell Birmingham, M.D., gave a check to Sister Mary Frances, who turned over the keys. Only part of the old hospital could be saved for modern use, however; the rest was demolished in a spectacular implosion. In 1977, the Progressive Care Center, designed for patients who required interim care, opened in a wing of the old hospital. An important later development was the construction of the crosswalk across Church Street that brought together the former Saint Thomas property and the original Baptist Hospital property. James H. Winters, chairman of the board, had felt for a number of years that this was a necessary construction project, and his dream was fulfilled when the crosswalk was completed in 1982. Since that time there have been two additional crosswalks—one across Twentieth Avenue and another across Twenty-first Avenue.

"I like working in the labor and delivery room because it's one of the most rewarding places in the hospital. . . . One of my greatest rewards is seeing those new parents with the new baby and smiling."
—*Christine Willis*

The 1980s marked a turning point in many ways. The public wanted big private rooms with baths for patients, and the hospital responded with the construction of the Kidd Building. More physicians desired to be closer to the hospital, thus more medical office buildings were planned as Baptist Medical Plaza I and II. The competition in health care called for more programs and services, which in turn meant more places to house them. The results were the Baptist Fitness Center, Outpatient Services, the Institute for Aesthetic and Reconstructive Surgery, and space for health and wellness programs.

Rev. Dr. Franklin Paschall, who served as board chairman from 1982 to 1988, remarked that Gene Kidd "was always a strong administrator and he had a good assistant in David Stringfield. We moved forward one building after another, and we closed out his term as president in 1981 with the new building named after him. That's a nice tribute to him." An even more aggressive building program was carried out while Stringfield was president and CEO.

Paul Moore summed up what has happened to the building program in the 1980s and beyond: "We thought when we did the first one, the $45 million expansion program [Kidd Building], we wouldn't have to do anything more for quite a while. But the growth of the hospital and the demand for services in the community grew to the extent that we are still building. I guess we always will be and that's a good situation to have."

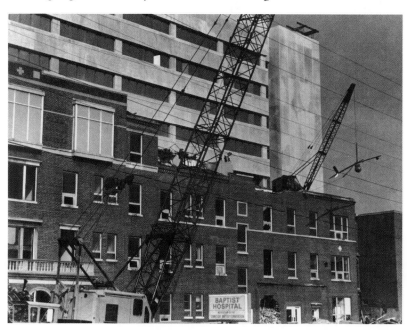

Construction—a common sight beginning in the 1980s.

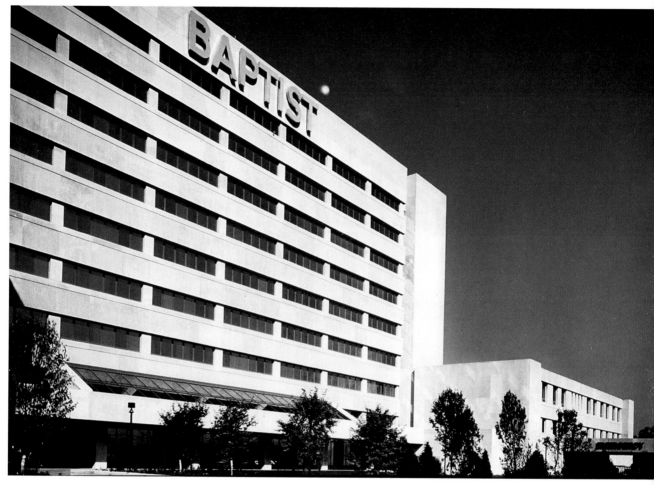

Kidd Building, 1984.

A brochure explained the $45 million construction and renovation to patients: "At Baptist Hospital, we have a philosophy that everything we do, every step we take, should ultimately benefit our patients in some way. When the final brick is laid in place, Baptist will have the newest, most up-to-date facility of any major hospital in Nashville." The building program goals included 398 private rooms; twenty-nine new obstetrical beds; enlarged radiology, lab, central supply, and pharmacy; the Intensive Care Unit consolidated in one unit; and a 580–foot elevated walkway over Church Street.

In August 1993, nine hundred people attended a celebration picnic held in the newest parking facility on Twentieth Avenue at State Street in honor of ten years of construction and expansion. On hand were employees, *local* construction workers, engineers, architects,

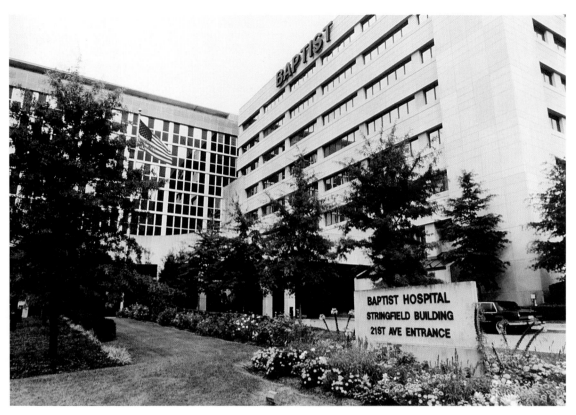

Stringfield Building, 1987.

subcontractors, and suppliers. Some of the firms included R. C. Mathews Contractor; Hart-Freeland-Roberts; Hardaway Construction; Gresham, Smith and Partners; Yearwood, Johnson, Stanton, and Crabtree; Earl Swenson Associates; and DWC Construction. Baptist Hospital takes pride in using local people on building projects. It is an another example of what the hospital does to contribute to the well-being of the community—this time, its financial well-being.

Through the building program from 1982 to 1998, nearly $500 million was invested in renovations, improvements, and new projects. During this period of growth, Gerald Hemmer, Baptist Hospital construction engineer, has had the job of preparing contracts for architects, designers, and contractors to be approved by the board, and overseeing all construction projects. Two particularly challenging parts of his job are getting everything concluded within the designated time frame—and usually before—and keeping up with the technological changes. For example, the completion of the Laser Center met an accelerated schedule, but technology had progressed to the point that even more changes had to be accommodated immediately.

The list of construction projects from 1983 to 1998 is extensive. The following reflects only the major projects (new construction as well as renovations):

1983   Physical Therapy Department

1984   Refaced South Building, Kidd Building

1985   Lithotripter Suite, Heliport, Baptist Medical Plaza I, Fitness Center, Outpatient Surgery Center

1987   C. David Stringfield Building

1988   Retrofitted Central Building, Labor/Delivery Renovation, Baptist Medical Plaza II

1989   Nashville Orthopedic Associates Building, Outpatient Surgery Addition, Wound Care Center

1990   South Building Diagnostic Pavilion, Laparoscopy and Laser Surgery Center, Outpatient Surgery Renovation

1991   222 Medical Office Building (Heritage), Twenty-first Avenue Parking Garage, Sleep Center

1993   Mid-State Medical Parking Garage, Twentieth Avenue Medical Office Building, Twentieth Avenue Parking Garage, Sports Medicine, MRI, The Institute for Aesthetic and Reconstructive Surgery

1994   Twentieth Avenue Nashville Medical Group, Twentieth Avenue Arthritis Care Center

"If you ever had a kidney stone, you know it hurts. It used to be surgery was the only way to remove them. . . . I came to Baptist Hospital where they have what they call the 'tools of progress'—a lithotripter to remove kidney stones without surgery. . . . I was home in one day."

                           —Everett Smith

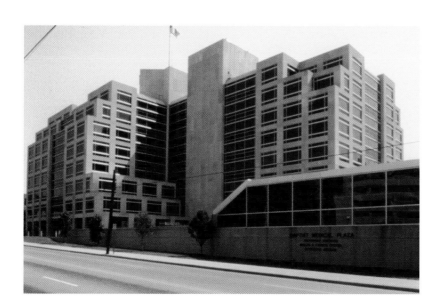

Baptist Medical Plaza I and II and the Fitness Center, 1985 and 1988.

1995   Gladys Stringfield Owen Education Center, Bellevue Medical Center Expansion, Early Morning Admission Unit

1996   PET Scan Suite

1997   Baptist Bellevue Renovation

1998   Heritage Mid-State Cardiology, Simulator Room, Endoscopy, North Medical Office Building, Baptist Ambulatory Surgery Center

The ground was broken in 1994 for the Gladys Stringfield Owen Education Center, a $4.1 million privately funded facility for community health and medical continuing education. It houses a teaching amphitheater, classrooms, and a comprehensive library for health professionals. Mrs. Owen's $1.5 million gift launched the fund-raising for the center. At the center's dedication in November 1995, Thomas G. Pennington, M.D., read the dedication statement: "We dedicate this new building to the worthy purposes of:

Educating the people of Middle Tennessee in maintaining good health,

Implosion of old Saint Thomas Hospital buildings.

Advancing the knowledge of physicians and other healthcare professionals,

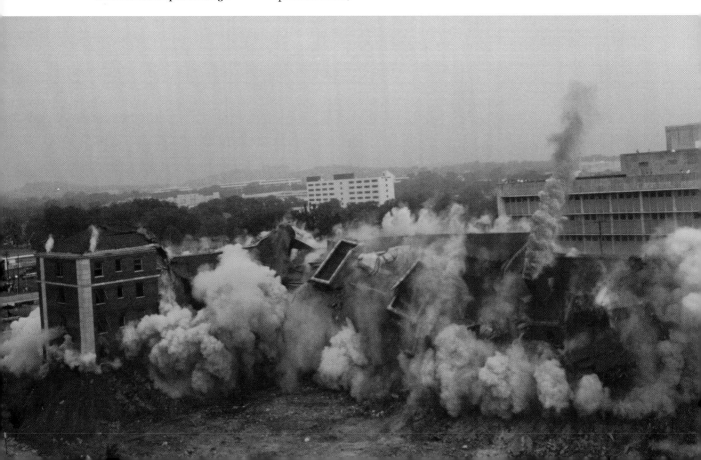

Serving as a permanent reservoir of health information, for the benefit of all,

Enhancing the reputation of Baptist Hospital and its healing ministry,

Contributing to the general welfare of the people of Nashville,

Serving as a lasting monument to the generosity of those whose donations made it a reality, and to the Glory of God."

The hospital main campus in 1998 covers more than six city blocks, with more than 1.5 million square feet. The hospital complex encompasses more than thirty-eight acres in more than fifty Davidson County locations. Here is a summary of the campus:

Central and South Buildings, both are eight stories with 327,000 square feet (ancillary and support services and patient care rooms)

Gene Kidd Building, nine stories with 170,000 square feet (ancillary and support services and patient care rooms)

Stringfield Building, eight stories with 133,000 square feet (ancillary and support services and patient care rooms)

Ford Building, three stories with 24,000 square feet (Emergency Pavilion and Cardiovascular Laboratory plus support and other services)

West Building, five stories with 58,000 square feet (ancillary support services, Residency Program, Center for Health and Wellness)

Mid-State Medical Center, seven stories with 113,000 square feet (medical offices for physicians, pharmacy, and Cancer Center)

Baptist Medical Plaza I and II, both are eight stories with 254,000 square feet (Outpatient Surgery, Outpatient Diagnostic Services, Institute for Aesthetic and Reconstructive

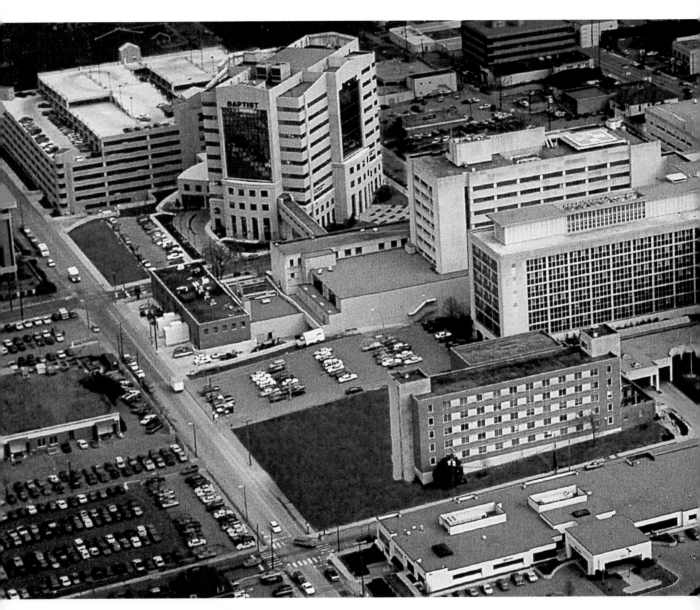

*Aerial view of Baptist Hospital
campus, 1994.*

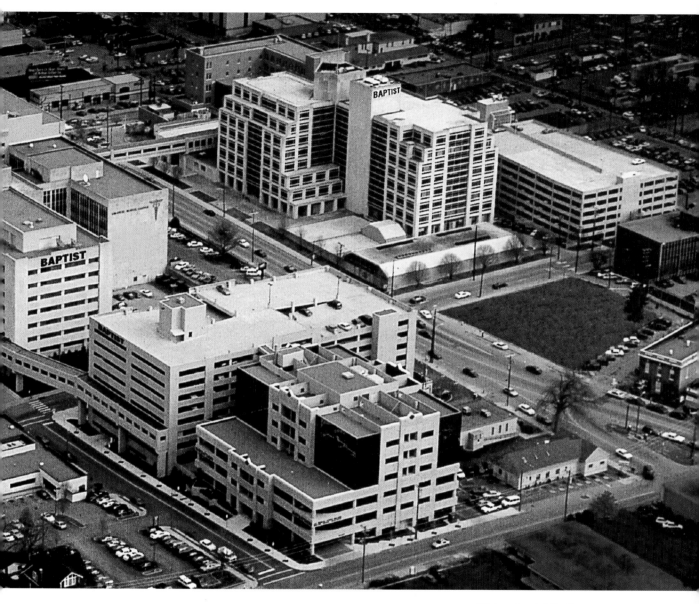

"Being stranded far from home, Oklahoma City, with a broken hip, I consider it my good fortune that Nashville was my 'downfall.'"
—Dr. & Mrs. Jay T. Shurley

Surgery, Health and Fitness Center, Sports Medicine Center, offices for forty-five physicians)

Rehabilitation Center, five stories with 74,000 square feet (rehab unit, subacute unit, pain management center, and other rehab services)

Gladys Stringfield Owen Education Center

Twenty-second Avenue Medical Office Building, six stories with 95,000 square feet

Twentieth Avenue Medical Office Building, nine stories with 279,000 square feet

Emergency Pavilion Expansion, 32,000 square feet (ER facility with six-bed chest pain center)

Ambulatory Surgery Center

North Medical Office Building, six stories with 161,760 square feet

Other convenient care clinics

"Thank you from the bottom of my heart for the compassion shown to me on Saturday, May 22, when I was so alone. I hope you know how much you helped. Also, please thank the CCU nurses who were kind way beyond the call of duty. I'm not sure I could have hung in there without you all. God bless you."

—Pat Duncan

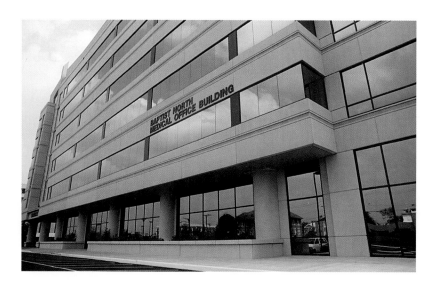

Baptist North Medical Office Building, 1998.

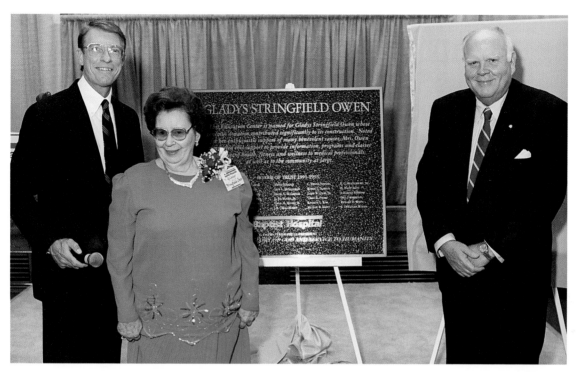

The dedication of the Gladys Stringfield Owen Education Center with David Stringfield, Gladys Stringfield Owen, and Governor Ned McWherter.

A vivid example of Baptist's ability to act rapidly and cooperatively on behalf of community health was the acquisition of the Middle Tennessee Medical Center in Murfreesboro. David Stringfield described how it happened: "For about a year I kept on hearing that the hospital may be sold to HCA. I knew the administrator very well, and I kept calling him and telling him, 'Please don't sell. Baptist Hospital could help with whatever your needs are.'

"I received a call one day at 3:00 P.M. from a very prominent person in Murfreesboro who said, 'If you don't do something, the hospital is going to be sold in the morning to HCA.' I knew that would necessitate many millions of dollars. I prayed about it. I said, 'Lord, guide me to what You want me to do.' I give the Lord credit for it. The Lord said to me, 'You [Baptist Hospital] and Saint Thomas are both well respected there. Why don't you do a joint venture—fifty-fifty—and acquire Murfreesboro Hospital?'

"I got our board's approval, and then I called the administrator at that time of Saint Thomas Hospital, Sister Juliana. I said, 'We have scheduled a press release for seven o'clock tonight, at which time Baptist Hospital will solely acquire the hospital or Saint Thomas can join with Baptist Hospital in a fifty-fifty joint venture.' She called back

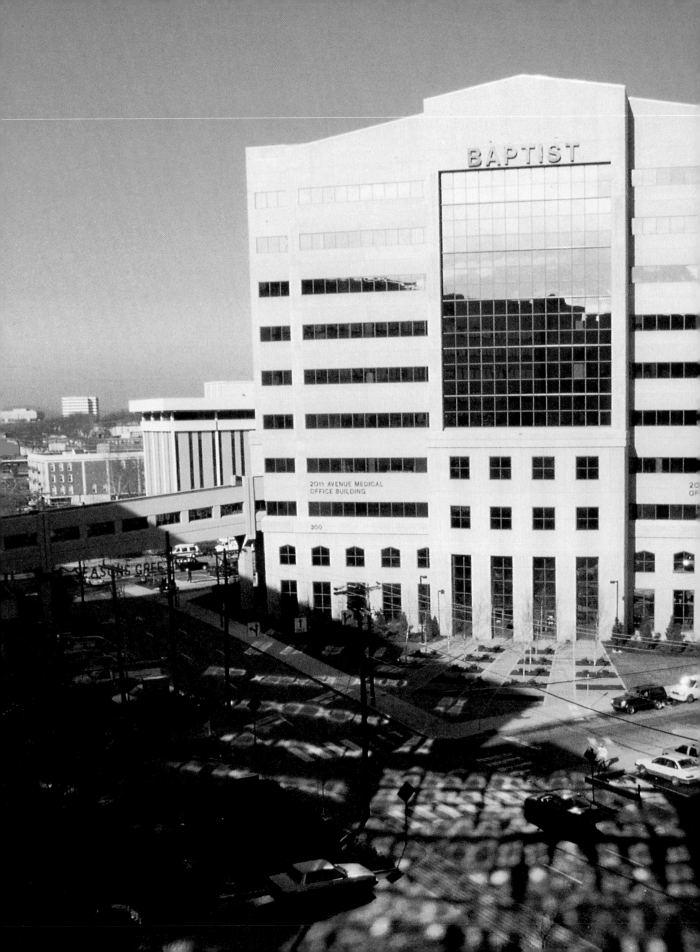

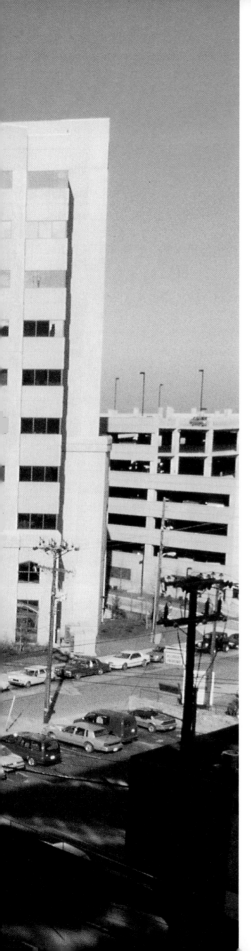

and said that they would participate in a fifty-fifty partnership.

"We had a press release at seven o'clock that night. Then we had to get our attorneys together to draft a written proposal. We had taxis and people deliver the written proposal to the trustees of the Murfreesboro Hospital at ten o'clock that same night.

"The proposal blocked the purchase by HCA. Some of the trustees of Murfreesboro Hospital said, 'We don't think that Baptists and Catholics can ever work together. Let's give them thirty days just to see if they can put the final deal together. We'd like to see a fight between the Baptists and the Catholics.' We never did have—and we never have had—any fights or arguments," said Stringfield.

"We [Baptist Hospital and Saint Thomas Hospital] initially told them that over a five-year period we would spend $10 million in capital improvements. We didn't spend $10 million. We spent $50 million. We've really improved the hospital there immeasurably. Since then we have spent even more than the $50 million in improvements. And the patient surveys have been quite favorable." Middle Tennessee Medical Center (MTMC) has a seventeen-member board, six representing the Daughters of Charity National Health System, six representing Baptist Hospital, and five local community leaders.

Twentieth Avenue Medical Office Building, 1993.

"On April 16, I delivered a baby boy at Baptist Hospital and I wanted to express my appreciation to the staff for making my stay a positive one. I also wanted to make you aware of the exceptional job that your staff members are doing. We appreciate the care that we received at Baptist Hospital, and because of our experience, we would choose your hospital again."
—Sheila Russell

Access has been Stringfield's theme of the 1990s. His ideas of taking services to where people live and work in this region spurred a period of expansion and acquisition. Baptist Hospital provides high-quality care to people in these locations: Baptist DeKalb Hospital in Smithville; Baptist Three Rivers Hospital in Waverly; Baptist Hickman Community Hospital in Centerville; Baptist Perry Community Hospital in Linden; Baptist-CentraCare Centers; Baptist Medical Plaza at Tennessee Christian Medical Center; Baptist Medical Center East in Hermitage; Baptist Convenient Care/WorkSmart on Elm Hill Pike; Baptist Physicians Pavilion Surgery Center on Wallace Road; Baptist Medical Center South on Harding Road; Cool Springs Family Clinic; Williamson/Baptist Medical Plaza at Cool Springs; Baptist Women's Pavilion South at Williamson Medical Center; Baptist Convenient Care Center in Murfreesboro; Ashland City Family Health Clinic; Occupational Medicine Center in Dickson; and Nolensville Family Care Center and Grassland Family Medical Center on Hillsboro Road, both projects of Williamson Baptist Medical Group.

Because of changes in health care and the emphasis on outpatient procedures and outpatient surgery, the future may not hold as many new large structures as have been built in the past. Although Baptist may stabilize at the present bed count, renovations of existing buildings and redefinitions of outpatient facilities guarantee a continuously active building program.

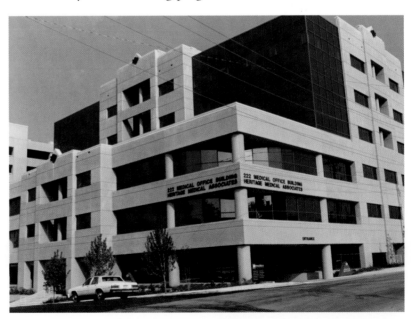

222 Medical Office Building, 1991.

Chapter 8

THE ACHIEVEMENTS OF A NOT-FOR-PROFIT HOSPITAL

Baptist has so many strengths, but its ability to be innovative is one of the most important.

—Paul W. Moore
Executive Vice President

"SHORTLY AFTER THE BAPTISTS ACQUIRED OWNERSHIP of the hospital, Mrs. Stow was to leave and many changes were beginning to take place under the administration of Mr. Robert M. Murphy, the new hospital administrator, and his bookkeeper, Miss Jamie Cheek.

"Nursing service was updated, and as a result more patients were being admitted to the hospital. New office equipment was acquired and soon the workload became too heavy for one cashier, so the second cashier was employed," recalled Mary E. Sesler, who was the hospital's cashier, then the insurance clerk, and last a secretary in Gene Kidd's office. Those were just the beginnings of changes, major and minor, in the hospital and health care.

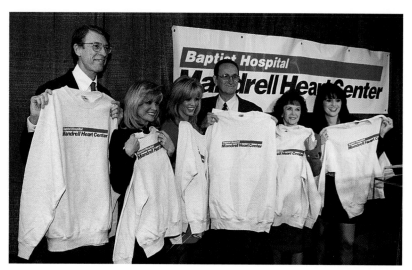

The Mandrell family has looked to Baptist Hospital for healthcare needs for three generations, notably for father Irby's heart condition. In honor of the long-standing relationship between the family and the hospital, the Mandrell Heart Center was dedicated in 1966. Left to right: David Stringfield, Barbara, Irlene, Irby, Mary, and Louise.

Administrators, staff, and board of Mid-State Baptist hospital had their work cut out for them with the limited programs and services in place in 1948, and to their credit, numerous improvements occurred within five years. However, improvements were gradual and on a fairly modest scale throughout the 1950s, 1960s, and 1970s.

The introduction of Medicare in July 1966 brought about challenges for the coming decades. At the same time the costs to run a hospital started increasing: complying with more and more governmental regulations (requiring time and personnel), keeping up-to-date medical technology, meeting energy needs, purchasing higher-priced malpractice insurance, dealing with costs of construction, offering fringe benefits for employees, and losing money in bad debts or community services.

Then a new venture in Nashville permanently altered the health-care picture. In 1962 Thomas F. Frist Sr., M.D., and five or six other physicians opened Parkview as a nursing home/hospital. A few years later Thomas Frist Jr. expressed interest in wanting to start a chain of for-profit hospitals. The idea was not new; it had been tried in California, but there were none in Tennessee. Frist Sr. and Frist Jr. and Jack Massey created Hospital Corporation of America (HCA) in 1969–70, sold stock, and went public with Parkview as the flagship hospital of the corporation. The physicians who had owned Parkview took stock in HCA as payment for their hospital. HCA set about buying other small hospitals and upgrading and improving them, first a few in rural Tennessee and Alabama, later in Virginia, Georgia, and other states.

The business community was skeptical about the new venture and its ability to become profitable—hospitals were not exactly known as big moneymakers—but because of Massey's involvement, business-people had to pay attention. Massey had sold his surgical supply company and enjoyed remarkable success with his investments in Kentucky Fried Chicken. Many people in the health community and the government disliked the for-profit hospital idea, and many accused HCA of profiting from the sick. By 1978, HCA encompassed more than one hundred hospitals, and it even had some international sites. When HCA merged with Columbia Healthcare Corporation in 1993, it became known as Columbia/HCA.

No matter what their feelings about HCA, most people would have to agree that the corporation is the reason for Nashville's becoming the corporate healthcare capital of the world. People copied the hospital idea with Hospital Affiliates, Humana, and dozens of others. Experienced and wealthy hospital executives who left HCA started peripheral operations in subspecialties of health care. By the end of the 1990s, Nashville was home to hundreds of these operations.

To keep up with the competitive healthcare environment in Nashville, Baptist Hospital had to expand services and attempt new ventures. President and CEO David Stringfield commented on the situation: "With the existence of for-profit hospitals, things are enormously more competitive."

A 1983 editorial in the *New England Journal of Medicine* presented this evaluation: "Judged not as businesses but as hospitals, which are supposed to serve the public interest, [for-profit hospitals] have been less cost-effective than their not-for-profit counterparts." The comments were based on three studies showing that for-profits were as much as 24 percent more expensive. Some average charges in the early 1980s reported by a BlueCross BlueShield-study indicated that Baptist had some of the lowest charges in the Middle Tennessee area: for a hernia, Baptist charged $1,109 whereas a for-profit charged $1,463; and for a heart attack, Baptist charged $2,337 whereas a for-profit charged $4,856.

Stringfield addressed the issue: "We are, by tradition and by choice, a humanitarian institution, more concerned with easing the suffering of our patients and the general health and well-being of the people of our community than with

"I think I appreciate life more now than ever. Four years ago while I was at work I had a numbness in my neck and within an hour and fifteen minutes I was completely paralyzed. I was rushed to Baptist Hospital. The encouragement I received in my seven weeks of rehabilitation at Baptist Hospital was a true blessing."
—Gerry Hunt

Country music superstar Louise Mandrell raised nearly half a million dollars at a Gala Dinner and Concert to benefit the Baptist Hospital Foundation. Here she presents a check to David Stringfield, President and CEO of Baptist. The funds were used to retire the debt for the Gladys Stringfield Owen Education Center.

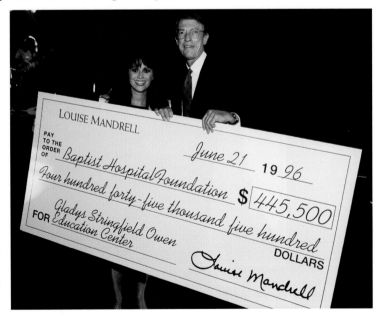

financial rewards. Our not-for-profit status makes that possible for us. Even so we recognize that to continue to serve Nashville and the surrounding area with high-quality health care, our hospital must be financially viable and able to keep operating and improving its services into the next century.

"We have achieved substantial savings through large-scale purchasing contracts, tight administrative controls on spending, and constant improvement in systems and procedures. We have involved our employees at all levels in identifying and implementing better ways to do things. Special teams of employees are constantly working on maximizing efficiency, better delivery of care, hospitalwide cost containment and greater productivity, with savings passed along to patients. Unlike for-profit hospitals, we are concentrating on output maximization for our patients and the community rather than profit maximization for shareholders in other areas."

The Hospital Alliance of Tennessee is a statewide association that was formed as a lobbying group on behalf of not-for-profit hospitals and the issues important to them. Stringfield was a founding board member, and Peaches Simpkins was also a founding board member and the first executive director of the group.

As a founding shareholder of Voluntary Hospitals of America, the nation's largest healthcare network, Baptist Hospital has joined about 1,200 not-for-profit health systems and hospitals to purchase supplies. Annual purchases have reached $11.3 billion for 1998, due in part to a merger this year with UHC (University Hospital Consortium). Baptist and thirty-four other hospitals began the centralized purchasing program to buy in large quantities with an economy of scale. It became a nationwide group, including major facilities, such as Johns Hopkins, Massachusetts General, and Cedars of Sinai, as well as smaller hospitals.

Baptist's financial stewardship has enabled the hospital to annually provide free services to the community, which include charity, unreimbursed patient costs (the major category here), and benefit programs. In 1993, for example, Baptist Hospital gave more than $43.9 million in total indigent care including uncompensated costs of government programs of $21 million, bad debt expense of $12.6 million, and charity/medically indigent care of $10.3 million. That figure represents about sixteen times as much charity/medically indigent care and about five times as much total indigent care as provided on average by Nashville's three top for-profit hospitals.

The increase in the total contribution, including all categories, over the years has been remarkable. In the 1950s it ranged from

The Baptist Emergency Pavilion, the busiest in Nashville, stands ready with highly trained personnel and state-of-the-art equipment 365 days and nights a year.

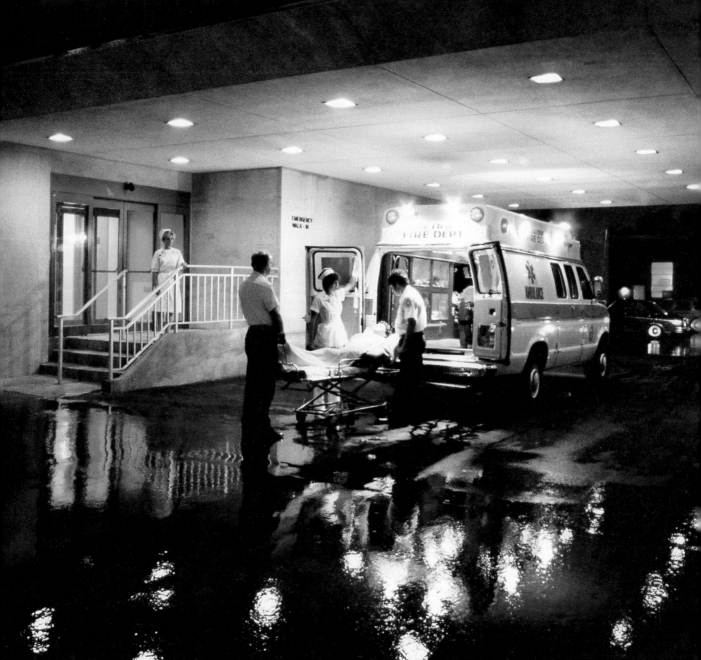

$50,000 to $170,000; in the 1960s it was in the $700,000s; in the 1970s it exploded from $1 million to more than $4 million; by the mid-1980s it rocketed up to $21 million; and it has been moving upward since then.

Baptist Hospital has earned a reputation for successfully implementing new programs. The vast majority of current programs and services have been started since 1982. How has the hospital done it? Stringfield highlighted flexibility as one component: "I really feel there are certain things that you can set certain deadlines on, but there are other things, such as the Lithotripter Center or the Laser Surgery Center, where you can't project advances in medicine. Therefore, you have to be in a position where you can be flexible and go with some of the latest and newest trends."

Paul Moore pointed out that "Baptist was the first hospital to do outpatient surgery in Nashville." The Short Stay Surgical Unit was established in July 1971. Later a new center was built in the Plaza complex. Moore continued, "We used to say we are spending money in order to save money. We are spending money so that the patients can come in and not have to stay overnight in the hospital. It was an idea whose time had come. The technology was available, the people were interested in saving money, and all of this happened to culminate at this particular point in time." Baptist's dedication to outpatient surgery has intensified, and the next century holds the likelihood of more of these procedures.

Baptist's programs and services have multiplied over the years as the needs of physicians and patients have been identified and acted upon.

Cardiac conditions continue to be major health concerns for Americans, and Baptist continues to work to help. The Mandrell Heart Center, dedicated in 1996, is staffed with registered nurses and nutritionists specializing in heart and vascular disease. It offers outpatient cardiac rehabilitation programs, including nutrition, exercise, stress management, and good health habits. There is a twenty-four-hour Chest Pain Hot Line. The cardiac imaging done in the PET Suite (PET is the Positron Emission Tomography scanner) has the goal of lowering risk and even reversing heart disease through noninvasive technology. UltraFast Imaging detects early stages of coronary artery disease.

The Women's Pavilion is designed to make having a baby a pleasant experience for the entire family.

For any person who requires emergency medical attention, the Baptist Emergency Pavilion is open twenty-four hours a day, 365 days a year. Donna Mason is the administrative director. With its physicians, nurses, and physician assistants who specialize in emergency care, the Emergency Pavilion has long been recognized as one of the finest emergency treatment centers in the Middle Tennessee region. It is the largest in the area in terms of volume of patients. The community's emergency needs have grown with the community: more than 9,000 visits in 1960, more than 24,000 in 1971, more than 37,000 in 1980, and more than 56,000 in 1990. In 1995 a redesigned pavilion opened, and the area includes private rooms, mobile equipment and supplies, computerization, and digital radiography. Opened in November 1997, the Chest Pain Observation Unit allows patients experiencing signs of a heart attack to have tests without being admitted to the hospital; it was the first of its kind in Middle Tennessee.

Women's health is the special concern of the Women's Pavilion and the Women's Pavilion Health Center. Baptist Women's Pavilion

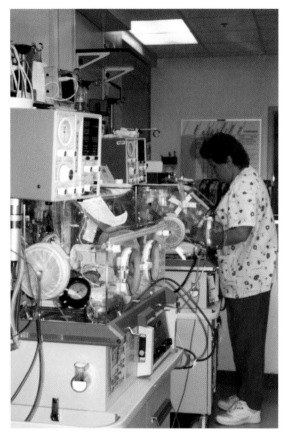

The Neonatal Intensive Care Unit just celebrated its twenty-second year of caring for the sickest and tiniest babies at Baptist.

opened in 1991. The Pavilion's community program includes initiatives aimed at promoting better women's health throughout Middle Tennessee: breast cancer awareness, prenatal care, parenting education, preteen education on body changes and self-esteem, and other related topics. Through the Breast Care Center, women have access to centralized breast evaluation and testing centers in addition to educational programs by the staff of the Women's Pavilion. A satellite mammography service, one of the first in the nation, was offered year-round at Castner Knott Department Stores in Green Hills Mall and in Bellevue Mall. Both locations were eventually closed because the volume was not great enough to make them financially viable. The equipment was moved downtown, and the staff was consolidated.

The staff at the Women's Pavilion gives new mothers the medical care they need, encourages family involvement, and provides support throughout the pregnancy and after the baby's birth. In addition to making provisions for labor rooms for traditional childbirth, the

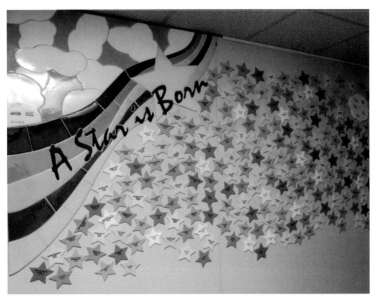

Proud parents can add a star in recognition of their child's birth to "A Star Is Born" wall in the Women's Pavilion.

Women's Pavilion has Labor/ Delivery/Recovery Suites that permit a family-centered birth experience and immediate availability of comprehensive obstetric services, if necessary. Mothers may choose to room-in, that is, have their newborns in their rooms rather than in the nursery.

Baptist Women's Pavilion Childbirth Education Classes inform attendees about planning for a healthy baby and give tips on health risks and lifestyle changes, and there are classes and seminars throughout the year. The popular Childbirth Fair is held once a year. The Pavilion launched a new program of education for pregnant teenagers in area high schools, in partnership with Crittenton Services.

A free service begun in 1998 was the Internet E-mail birth announcement. A staff member photographs the newborn with a digital camera, and the parents receive a disc to use in the Pavilion's computer terminal and Internet connection to compose and send a message. It is not a Web site, so it is more personal and secure.

Women's Pavilion Health Center, staffed with specially trained nurse educators, is for women beyond their childbearing years. Among the services are programs on topics ranging from menopause to midlife crisis, individual health risk appraisals, and private counseling on issues including nutrition, hormone replacement therapy, osteoporosis prevention, cardiovascular health, breast care, female cancer, and hysterectomy. Mammography screenings are available. The Resource Library offers videos, books, and pamphlets. Through the speaker's bureau, qualified speakers may be scheduled for civic and community groups to address topics related to women's health care.

Baptist Hospital has been a leader in offering advanced technology to improve patient care, and these centers are excellent examples. The Laparoscopy and Laser Surgery Center (today called the Laparascopy Center) was the first facility in the nation to be designed for, equipped, specifically staffed, and dedicated solely to laparoscopic and laser surgery for the treatment of gynecological disorders, such as the removal of ovarian cysts and fibroid tumors, and the treatment of abdominal disorders, such as those affecting the gall-bladder; other procedures include hysterectomies, appendectomies, and hernia repairs. Baptist Stone Treatment Center is the home of Middle Tennessee's first lithotripter. It now has two of the devices to eliminate kidney stones without surgery. Of note is that Baptist Hospital was one of five testing centers for the fifth-generation lithotripter. Baptist urologists submitted more than half of all the cases from those five centers sent to the Food and Drug Administration to secure approval for its use.

Recognizing the trend toward more outpatient procedures, Baptist Hospital opened the Early Morning Admission (EMA) Unit in 1995. It was the nation's first specially constructed, self-contained unit of its type. The forty-one-bed unit, covering 24,000 square feet, is a one-stop facility that serves as a preadmission testing and preoperative unit for patients scheduled for surgery, as well as a postoperative unit for patients who have same-day surgery in the main hospital operating suites. In addition, it serves as an overnight courtesy floor for surgery patients who have early morning procedures scheduled or who live outside Nashville. The unit is fully staffed

"Like most first-time mothers I didn't know what to expect. I've always heard that Baptist Hospital was the place to go to have a baby. I went to the baby birthing classes and my fears were gone and I got very excited."
—Michelle Hawn

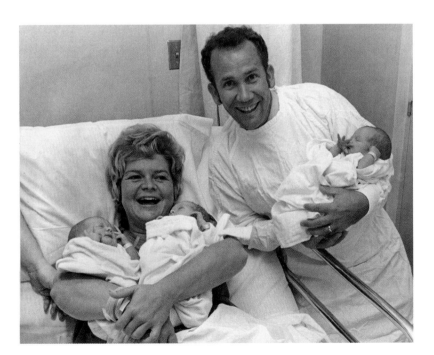

Triplets may prove to be a handful for parents, but the staff at the Women's Pavilion is prepared to help parents before and after their arrival.

and equipped for lab and diagnostic testing, and anesthesia consultation and nursing assessments are done on site.

The free-standing Outpatient Surgery Center is another response to meet the growing need for outpatient procedures. It offers same-day surgery and diagnostic testing; a full range of medical imaging, using the area's most powerful MRI equipment; mammography; a full-service radiation oncology unit; thirty-seven private preoperative and postoperative rooms; and fourteen operating suites. In the 1950s same-day surgery was unheard of; in 1951, there were more than 3,000 surgeries at Baptist; in the mid-1960s, there were more than 8,000 surgeries; in 1984, there were 1,733 short-stay surgeries and 13,689 surgeries in the main operating rooms; in 1990, there were 9,129 short-stay surgeries, 13,607 surgeries in the main operating rooms, and 87,338 outpatient registrations (includes diagnostic and therapeutic services such as MRI, CT scan, cardiac catheterization, dialysis, and lab services); in 1997, outpatient registrations were 268,456, and there were 10,748 surgeries in the main operating rooms but 16,491 in the Plaza, Laser Suite, the Institute for Aesthetic and Reconstructive Surgery, and Lithotripter Center.

Specific centers care for persons with specific conditions. Cancer patients and their families come to Baptist Cancer Center for individualized, personal attention and care. Specially trained nurses, nutritionists, and social workers work one-on-one with patients. An enterostomal therapist works with patients who have colostomies and ileostomies. In March 1995 the center was accredited by the Commission on Cancer of the American College of Surgeons. Baptist Hospital pursued the voluntary accreditation. Specialized programs include the Radiation Oncology Program, the Tumor Registry, and the Bone Marrow Transplant Program.

Baptist Stroke Center, part of the Neuroscience Center, is dedicated to acute and long-term care of stroke patients. Several specialists have been added, for example, in neuroradiological diagnostic and interventional therapies. It opened in November 1995.

Physicians in the Baptist Arthritis and Osteoporosis Care Center diagnose and treat arthritis, osteoporosis, and other related rheumatic diseases; specialized counseling is available for patients and families.

Baptist Diabetes Center deals with diabetes management and education. Programs in nutrition, insulin pump use, ambulatory insulin injections, and gestational diabetes complement physician care.

Baptist Wound Care Center is one of only a few in the United States, and the only one in Middle Tennessee. Nonhealing wounds

"I was a patient at Baptist and was treated like royalty and I just wanted to let you know how nice everybody was. I can't single out any one person because you all were very caring. I had a double by-pass. I want to thank you all for your kindness. It's nice to know you don't have to be a top name to get the best service there is!"

—*Sunshine Hay*

caused by diabetes, pressure sores, peripheral vascular disease, and so on are treated with a solution created from growth factors extracted from the patient's blood.

The laboratory is an integral part of the healthcare services. In Baptist LabPlus, standard lab work, from testing for pregnancy to testing glucose levels, can be done in a location convenient for the patient. It opened in October 1995. LabPlus is a reference lab for numerous clinical labs within physicians' offices, nursing homes, clinics, and other hospitals. Its success stems from the attention to its clients' need, its high-quality service, and its cost-competitiveness.

Baptist Hospital Rehabilitation Services include inpatient rehabilitation programs for head injuries, spinal cord injuries, strokes, respiratory problems, and other physical disabilities. Other rehabilitation services on both inpatient and outpatient bases include acute care, pediatric rehabilitation, and hand and musculoskeletal services. Baptist WorkSmart Center for Industrial Rehabilitation aims to return workers to the job after an injury and to work with industry to prevent injuries.

The Subacute Unit, located in the Rehabilitation Center, is designed for patients in a recovery stage between needing acute care and being ready to go home, such as patients who have had joints replaced or who have had extensive illnesses. The unit opened in January 1996 with thirty-six beds, but the immediate need for more beds resulted in the addition of eighteen more not long afterward. The average length of stay is two weeks, with some patients staying only one week but others staying as long as eight weeks. Each patient's physician works with a team of healthcare professionals.

At The Institute for Aesthetic and Reconstructive Surgery, opened in 1990, internationally known physicians perform a wide range of plastic and reconstructive surgeries. Some patients may benefit from professional medical makeup and camouflaging consultation. The Craniofacial Restoration Unit (plastic surgeons and specialists in ophthalmology, oral surgery, and pediatrics) restores a more normal appearance to individuals with deformities of the skull and face as a result of birth anomalies, cancer, or trauma. Through the marvels of computer imaging, individuals may visualize how cosmetic surgery can change their appearance. The Hair Restoration Unit is equipped for surgical and nonsurgical treatments for baldness, including micro- and minigrafts. In 1998, the Aesthetic Laser Center opened with the look and feel of a spa. Plastic surgeons trained in laser technology treat acne scars, age/sun spots, birthmarks, rosacea, scars, stretch marks, and tattoos.

"I was fortunate, I came to Baptist Hospital where they have a machine called a lithotripter. If you've ever had a kidney stone you know how much it hurts. It used to be that surgery was the only way to get rid of them. There's a real professionalism at Baptist that I don't believe you'll find anywhere else."
—Everett Smith

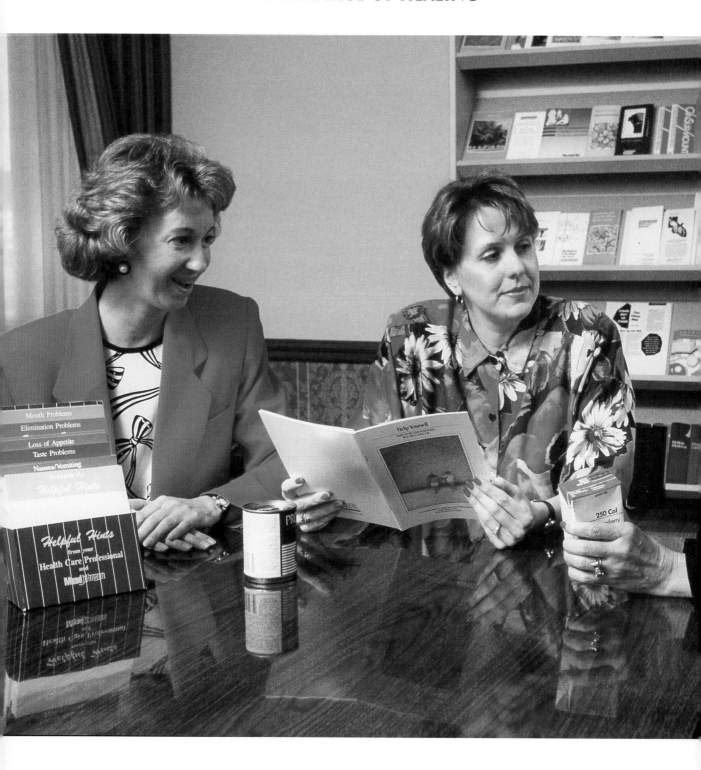

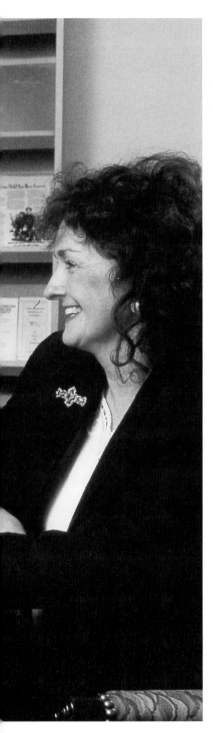

The Institute is a nationwide resource center for public and professional education. Baptist Hospital hosted the world's largest gathering of plastic surgeons specializing in reconstructive aesthetic breast surgery in May 1995. For its second symposium, Baptist Hospital was cosponsor with Baptist Center for Medical Education. On the occasion David Stringfield remarked, "Our mission to educate the community reaches beyond state and even national boundaries, and we are honored to have the opportunity to share our expertise on an international level." Attending were more than one hundred physicians from Brazil, Denmark, England, France, Germany, Italy, Mexico, Saudi Arabia, Sweden, Switzerland, Russia, and Turkey. The medical director of the Institute is G. Patrick Maxwell, M.D. The Institute reached out to the community with its services by offering free surgery and postoperative care to Operation Smile U.S.A., a group providing surgical assistance to children with facial deformities.

Patients who go to the Baptist Sleep Center benefit from a state-of-the-art lab and experienced staff specially trained in evaluating and treating sleep disorders, such as sleep apnea, narcolepsy, and insomnia. It is accredited by the American Sleep Disorders Association, a voluntary organization to establish standards for sleep centers in the United States.

Baptist Mind/Body Medical Institute is an affiliate of Harvard Medical School and Beth Israel/Deaconess Hospital. The approach is to improve patient health by changing lifestyles and emotional

The Baptist Cancer Center provides comprehensive services including nutritional counseling.

responses, and developing positive human outlooks to augment traditional medical treatment. It uses relaxation techniques and other self-help methods to treat disorders caused or worsened by stress. Modern medicine, psychology, and nursing are integrated with nonpharmacologic treatments to strengthen the natural healing capabilities of mind and body. Pain management, medical symptom reduction (outpatient clinic for chronic illness or stress-related physical symptoms, such as headaches, back pain, gastrointestinal problems, skin problems, pain syndromes, anxiety, sleep disorders, fatigue, asthma, allergies), cardiac rehabilitation, and insomnia are targets of the program.

Baptist Allergy Center's pollen-mold hot line is the only facility in the region that monitors the daily pollen and mold spore counts in the county. The information is used by the local media to alert the public and by Baptist physicians to prepare allergy medications for their patients. The data are shared with a nationwide data-gathering center to assist patients with known allergies relative to a good place for them to live as allergy-free as possible. The center also offers seminars about types, causes, and treatment of allergies.

Baptist Hospital recognizes the spiritual as well as the physical needs of patients. To better serve patients and their families, the Department of Pastoral Services has two full-time chaplains. The twenty-five to thirty volunteers who are retired clergypersons or laypersons visit all of the patients.

Lewis Lamberth, Director of Pastoral Services, has been at Baptist Hospital for eighteen years, and he has been in chaplain service all of his career. He said, "I get paid to help people and do what I love to do—what can be better than that?" He described several functions of his department:

The chaplains minister to needs of patients and family members in the role of pastoral counselor. They deal with critical news to patients and people in crisis situations. A big change Lamberth has observed is that they had a longer time to get to know patients in the past; now patients are in and out of the hospital almost overnight. For personal, marital, and grief counseling, people come to the pastoral office for scheduled sessions.

The chaplains administer Communion, and they may baptize by immersion or sprinkling, whatever is possible when requested.

The chaplains hold a worship service each Wednesday at noon for twenty minutes, broadcast over closed-circuit TV in the hospital.

The chaplains officiate at weddings—mainly for staff—and at funeral or memorial services.

"I just can't say enough about what a wonderful experience I had at Baptist. The room was great. All the nurses were so friendly. I had the best experience in Labor and Delivery. I'd choose Baptist in a minute all over again!"
—*Heather Schmidt*

The chaplains have most recently been involved in spirituality study groups of Baptist employees, emphasizing spirituality in the workplace. The immediate impetus was Sir John Templeton's book on spiritual principles and his visit to Nashville. Spirituality and the whole-person emphasis reflect changes and hunger for such in society. And now corporate America is recognizing and responding to the need.

Any effort by the department is a ministry. Lamberth explained that the "basic relationship is between you and the patient and God." That goes beyond theology to get to the real thing. He viewed his job as being a "representative of God," a humbling job assignment.

As part of its long-term strategy to take health care to the people, where they live or work, Baptist Hospital established several operations within its Baptist Affiliates organization. These include Baptist Healthcare Group (BHG), which owns and manages clinics, family health centers, and physicians' offices at multiple locations throughout greater Nashville and the Middle Tennessee area. More than fifty physicians practice at one of these locations, conveniently situated in small towns and metropolitan neighborhoods across the area.

BHG was the first fully integrated healthcare model in the state of Tennessee, when it was formed by the hospital in 1993. Physicians practice in a number of specialties, including family medicine, pediatrics, obstetrics and gynecology, internal medicine, dermatology, and others.

Baptist also established Baptist Convenient Care, which operates walk-in clinics at several locations in the Nashville area, offering physician services on weekends and extended weekday hours for the convenience of patients needing immediate and unscheduled health care. Lab and X-ray services, school and sports physicals, corporate physicals, and occupational health programs are also available.

Baptist Hospital Home Health provides residential nursing care to homebound patients in more than twenty Middle Tennessee counties from offices in Nashville, Clarksville, Franklin, Lebanon, and Lewisburg. The program was founded by Joanne Knight, and the hospital purchased it from her. Knight went on to become a vice president on Baptist's Administrative Staff with responsibility for Home Health as well as a number of other departments. "Mother's Helper" programs assist mothers with newborn and older children. The hospital's Medicare-certified home care affiliate provides skilled nursing visits, home health aide visits, and therapy and social service visits. The private duty nursing home care agency provides skilled nursing care as well as companion care. These services aid patients who seek alternative living arrangements and seniors who need

"I just want you to know how I feel about one of your marvelous Home Care nurses. Never have I known such a wonderful, dedicated person. I feel perfectly safe in her hands and if there's a chance of me getting better sooner, she's the one who can do it."

—Carolyn Carver

intermittent as well as twenty-four-hour services. There are therapeutic services in the home—physical, speech, and occupational. And there are infusion services—chemotherapy, pain management, and fluid replacement. In 1993, Baptist Hospital Home Health was accredited with commendation by the Joint Commission on Accreditation of Healthcare Organizations.

An adjunct to Home Health is Baptist Medical Equipment and Supplies, which provides needed equipment to the residential patients as well as disposable supplies. This is an important factor in providing health care in the home.

All of these outreach programs are offered by Baptist Hospital to make health care more convenient and affordable for patients and their families, and to assure that Baptist quality care is available at locations easily accessible to everyone in Middle Tennessee.

Four Occupational Medicine Centers help companies better manage healthcare costs by improving and supporting workers' compensation programs, organizing medical care for injuries on the job, and providing regulatory support. Services include workers' compensation cost reduction analysis; internal case management support; medical care, assessment, consultation, and physical examinations for workers' compensation injuries; ADA-90 compliance; drug screening; and program development. In 1994, for example, the centers served 26,953 patients.

Baptist Hospital's Early Morning Admissions Unit has been a unique response to the growing demand for ways to accommodate outpatient procedures. Among those participating in the EMA opening were left to right: Dr. John Tudor, Evelyn Springer, Dr. John Dalton, Shirley Johnson, and Paul Moore.

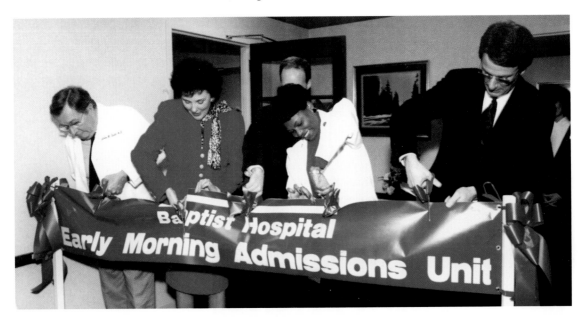

CompPlus, formed by Baptist, is a managed care organization specifically developed to address workers' compensation injuries. It combines a comprehensive provider network with a managed care product designed to lower employers' healthcare costs. Medical protocols, billing, and communications systems are customized to meet the needs of each company.

Baptist Hospital founded Health Net Management, Inc., in 1984 as the region's first independent PPO, and it has now grown to be the largest, with 235,650 persons covered. It includes HMO, PPO, PPO Plus, HMO POS/Health Net 65 (a Medicare product), ASO, and TPA services. (Some explanation of terms may be helpful. An HMO [Health Maintenance Organization] is set up with emphasis on maintenance; the goal is to provide early treatment and prevent major illnesses, thus keeping costs down. HMOs represent capitated insurance plans in which individuals or their employers pay a fixed monthly fee. In a PPO [Preferred Provider Organization], the individual or the employer receives a discounted rate if a doctor is among a preselected group; if a doctor is outside the PPO, the individual pays more out of pocket. ASO refers to administrative services only. TPA refers to a third-party administrator.) A feature of Health Net's success is the unique composition of its board, which includes physicians, business leaders, and others from the community in equal numbers of four for each category.

The EAR (Education and Auditory Research) Foundation at Baptist Hospital is a not-for-profit foundation to advance education and auditory research. Community educational and support programs are available for hearing and balance-impaired individuals. Baptist underwrites and provides free space for the foundation. In addition to support from the hospital, the EAR Foundation is supported with proceeds from the annual Balloon Classic in Nashville.

The Baptist Hospital Foundation is a nonprofit organization established to provide and enhance patient care services and further the goals of the hospital through the acquisition of new buildings, resource materials, and equipment through private donations. The contributions are tax deductible and can be made in the form of cash, securities, real property, and other assets. Before the formation of the foundation, no mechanism was in place if someone wanted to donate money to be

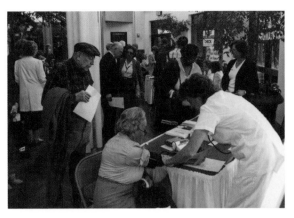

The hospital sponsors many events each year to promote wellness within the community.

used to benefit the hospital, according to Art Victorine, senior vice president of external affairs.

In 1991, the foundation dedicated "A Star Is Born" Baby Wall of Fame. Artist David Wright handcrafts a ceramic star in a pastel color with the baby's name and birth date. The $100 contribution for the star goes to Baptist Hospital Foundation. All of the stars are displayed on a wall near the nursery in the Women's Pavilion, and there are a few clouds with families of several children.

The funds for the Gladys Stringfield Owen Education Center came through the foundation. Mrs. Owen was raised in Monterey, educated in Nashville and Crossville, and received her nursing degree from Nashville General Hospital. The initial funding for the Education Center came from Mrs. Owen. In 1996 Louise Mandrell organized "A Tribute to Baptist Hospital," a spectacular fund-raiser that brought in a net of more than $400,000 and completed funding for the Education Center. Country superstar Crystal Gayle entertained guests at the 1998 event. The foundation also raises money with a holiday shopping party at Crystal's in Belle Meade Plaza each year and through donations from employees, physicians, and the general public.

All of these departments and services exist at Baptist Hospital only to reinforce the commitment to quality health care to the community. The staff, the administrators, and the Board of Trustees have met this commitment in the past and in the present and will continue efforts to meet it in the future.

Chapter 9

COMMUNITY OUTREACH

*We focus on ways to help people learn to stay healthy
and hopefully out of the hospital.*
—Willa Manchester
Director, Center for Health and Wellness

AT THE TURN OF THE TWENTIETH CENTURY, infectious diseases caused most illnesses. Then came better sanitation, immunizations, and antibiotics. Heart disease, cancer, stroke, and accidents have taken the places of infectious diseases as serious health threats to Americans. The cost of treating all illnesses has risen precipitously: $41 billion in 1965, more than $130 billion in 1975, $428 billion in 1985, and $988 billion in 1995, according to the U.S. Department of Health and Human Services. But each individual *can* do something about these rising costs, and Baptist Hospital has been ahead of the times in responding to this need and preparing for the next century of health care.

Addie Hamilton pointed out an important development in Baptist Hospital's services: "The development of the educational programs for the community, from how to care for diabetic patients to how to bathe a baby to how grandparents can help with a new baby to sports medicine and exercise therapy." She emphasized that people should be more knowledgeable about their health care and ways to maintain their health, and one of the hospital's major roles in the future will be to provide more opportunities for them to gain this information.

Baptist Hospital began many such programs in the early 1980s and currently sponsors more than nine hundred free community classes and seminars; tens of thousands of people have attended them each of the past few years. Most are part of the LiveSmart Community Education Classes and screenings. No matter what the program, the focus is on the maintenance of a healthy lifestyle.

Events and Support Groups

The hospital's Calendar of Events is full year-round. Every provision is made to schedule programs at times convenient to the most people who can benefit from them. Women may take the Childbirth Refresher Course, the Breastfeeding Class, the Prenatal and Postpartum Water Exercise Class, and the Early Pregnancy Class. The Arthritis Water Class, Tai Chi Chuan, and AARP Driving Seminar are suitable for older people. General classes include Tai Kwon Do, Yoga, CPR for Healthcare Providers, Pediatric CPR, Brothers and

Irlene Mandrell served as honorary chairman of Baptist's "Dance for Heart" at the Health and Fitness Center.

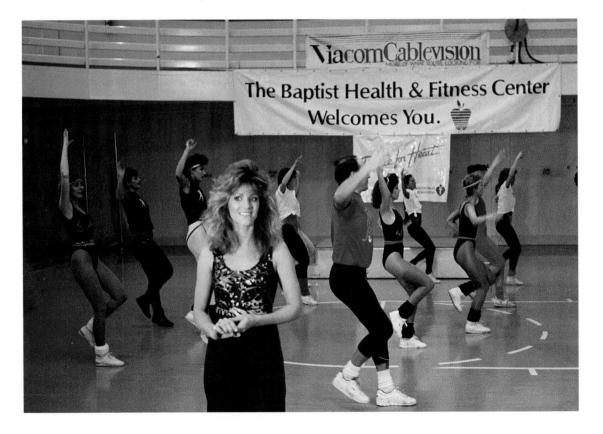

Sisters-to-be Class, Step, and Slide & Sculpt. Living Well with Diabetes and the Arthritis and Hip Pain Seminar are for people with more specific health problems. And these are only samplings of the available programs.

Several support groups hold regular meetings at the hospital: Breast Concerns and Mastectomy, Second Wind (for chronic pulmonary diseases), Impotents Anonymous, Tough Love, Cocaine Anonymous, Alcoholics Anonymous, Al-Anon, Cancer Support Group, US TOO (for prostate cancer patients), Neurofibromatosis Chapter, and a Bereavement Support Group are among them.

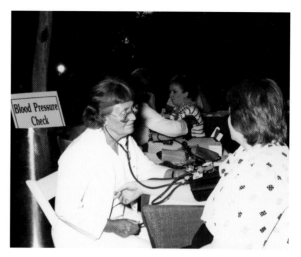

Baptist's communitywide blood pressure screenings prove valuable in alerting people to a serious health threat.

Health and Wellness

Baptist Hospital has an entire department dedicated to the prevention and early detection of disease to keep people out of the hospital. The Center for Health and Wellness arranges for educational classes for the community as well as health screenings, fitness testing, physicals for executives, and other work-site wellness programs for businesses and organizations. On-site programs include group CPR classes; educational classes on topics such as first aid, stress management, nutrition, and exercise; screenings for blood pressure, cholesterol, and physical fitness; health risk appraisals; and flu shots and hepatitis B vaccinations. SmokeBusters is one of the most successful smoking cessation programs in the region. Other programs include instruction in the basics of healthy nutrition; The Solution, a permanent weight loss program; and a children's weight management program.

Offered through the Baptist Mind/Body Medical Institute, Success Over Stress (SOS) is a program with a physician, a psychologist, and an exercise physiologist. Most people experience fifty or more stress events *per day*, although our bodies are designed to handle three or four events *per week*. Therefore, we need to recognize and manage our reactions to stress, and this program can help.

One of the more innovative programs, held in early June 1998, deserved mention in an article by Ray Waddle in *The Tennessean*. The hospital considers spiritual wellness a big part of the overall wellness picture. Sir John Templeton, the founder of the Wall Street Templeton

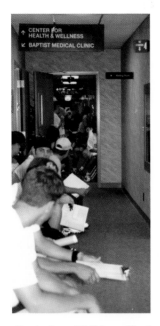

Baptist Sports Medicine staff and physicians provide free sports screenings for nearly four thousand middle and high school student athletes each year.

Funds and a Winchester, Tennessee, native, has written numerous books; among them is *Worldwide Laws of Life*, which "summarizes 200 spiritual principles boiled down from the world's fund of faith and folk wisdom." Baptist Hospital staff members studied the book as the "first known workplace pilot program for Templeton's vision." Templeton's campaign is to raise the quality of spiritual life in the United States. Baptist Hospital President David Stringfield said "the Templeton book study groups have been the best morale-builder I have seen in my thirty years here. I hope that other corporations will follow the example set by Baptist Hospital, for it will make for a more satisfied patient-customer and employee."

Seniors

Senior citizens and people nearing their senior years deserve special programs. The CareLine Emergency Response for Seniors is a personal emergency telephone response system offered to seniors or persons living alone or at risk. The 55PLUS free senior program began in 1987 and held its first 55PLUS Expo in June 1988. Ten years later, it has 80,000 members. The benefits include free membership, free classes and seminars on health-related topics, complimentary and discounted hospital services, and discounts from area merchants. Its InfoLine is open twenty-four hours a day with information on trips, events, seminars, and health fairs. On a recent trip arranged through 55PLUS, forty-four people went to Australia and New Zealand.

Baptist sponsors many communitywide events to promote good health and wellness, including the annual Baptist Fitness Race held each April.

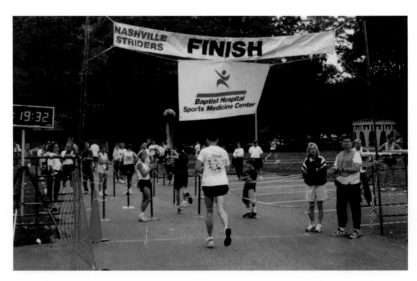

Physicians and Nurses

CareFinders is a free physician referral service, started in 1985, the first such program in the region. Baptist Nurse On Call was started in 1995, and with the help of a computer medical data system, registered nurses recommend physician-approved treatments for minor medical problems. They also advise when to see a doctor or go to the emergency department. The nurses have specific experience in critical care, emergency care, and pediatrics.

Cardiac Care

Because of the high numbers of Americans with cardiac problems, cardiac care is a prominent part of the hospital's outreach to the

Baptist employees teamed up to win the Corporate Challenge trophy for five consecutive years.

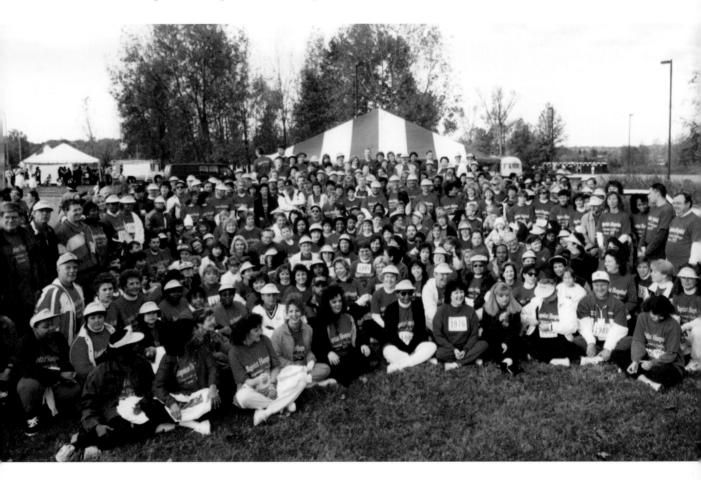

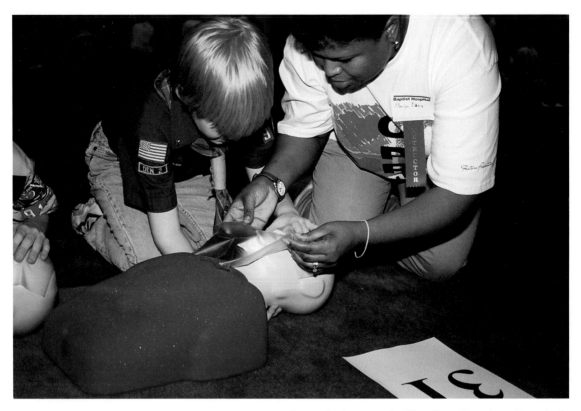

CPR instruction can save lives, and Baptist Hospital, WSMV-TV, and the Red Cross have sponsored communitywide efforts to train as many people as possible.

community. Coordinated in Nashville by Baptist Hospital, CountDown USA in 1988 was the first national screening for cholesterol and blood pressure. Of the 3,000 attendees, 65 percent were found to have borderline or high cholesterol, and 16 percent had high blood pressure. A 1994 Heart Smart Screening, in which 1,555 people got a health risk appraisal, discovered 51 percent at risk for high blood pressure and 60 percent at risk for high cholesterol. Another significant 1994 event was the Healthy Choice American Heart Walk with 700 participants, which raised $43,000. From 1993 to 1997 Baptist Hospital, as its major sponsor, participated with other community groups in the walk that funds American Heart Association research and community education programs. Baptist staff members have worked to train Middle Tennesseans in cardiopulmonary resuscitation (CPR). In 1997 more than 3,600 people participated in CPR Saturday events, cosponsored with the American Red Cross and WSMV-TV-Channel 4; the campaign was launched at the Nashville Convention Center with 1,200 participants.

Leadership

The Caduceus Society for Young Leaders was organized to give young Nashville leaders an opportunity to learn more about the area's vital health issues and share ideas with Baptist Hospital executives and physicians. Membership is by invitation each year. The list of speakers for the group has been impressive: in 1993, Lamar Alexander; in 1994, former U.S. Secretary of State Lawrence Eagleburger; in 1995, Tennessee Commissioner of Finance and Administration Robert Corker; and in 1996, Mike McClure, executive vice president of administration for the Oilers football team.

Volunteers

Through the Department of Volunteer Services, individuals offer their skills and time to Baptist Hospital. Perhaps it could be called community "inreach." Many volunteers are involved because they have been patients and want to give back for the care and services they have received.

Volunteers have given of themselves throughout the hospital's long history, but an official organization was formed in May 1965. The first annual membership meeting was held February 17, 1966, with Mrs. Douglas Shotwell presiding. One of the group's significant early achievements was financing the decoration of the hospital's Pediatric Playroom with proceeds of their daily coffee service. The opening of the playroom, which was for all patients under age twelve, was coordinated with the celebration of the hospital's Twentieth Anniversary Week.

Four types of volunteers can be found in the hospital. The Pink Ladies pay dues to belong to the organization, and they sell coffee and newspapers to raise funds for scholarships for the nursing program through Nursing Education. Junior Volunteers, no longer called Candystripers because the boys

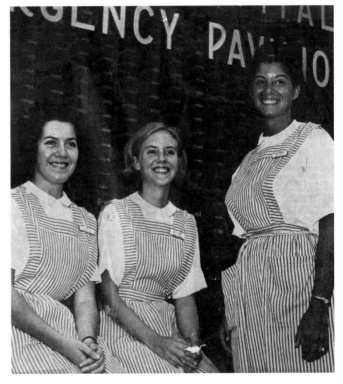

Candystripers were a common sight at one time as young women volunteered their time to the hospital; today the hospital's Junior Volunteers program attracts many young men and women each summer.

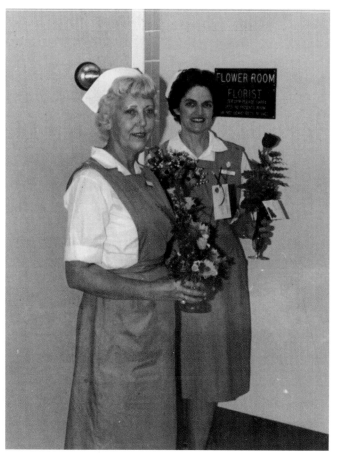

*Delivering flowers is only one
of many volunteer activities
at Baptist.*

objected, are fourteen to eighteen years old; girls wear pink smocks and boys wear blue jackets. Members of the Auxiliary, made up of women from the churches, especially the Women's Missionary Union, knit and crochet items for babies and supply magazines as well as other items used by patients and families. Other volunteers are usually available for shorter terms than people in the other categories. A volunteer may choose from among these tasks: clerical, rehab, social services, pastoral, nursing, admitting, Emergency Pavilion, ArthritisCare Center, Coronary Care Unit, and hostess cart. Junior Volunteers help with work in the lab, admitting, medical imaging, ArthritisCare, and other areas. Volunteers often join paid staff members at the information desks, which are open seven days a week.

A luncheon held once a year during National Volunteer Week honors volunteers for their hours of service. In 1968, 207 Candystripers gave 30,000 hours, and more than 200 women volunteers gave 18,000 hours. Three women who received 1,000–hour pins in 1968 were Mrs. Leo Newman, Mrs. Chester Jones, and Mrs. J. W. Fort. In 1992, there were 400 volunteers with 31,467 hours. Gladys Kittrell was recognized in 1997 for delivering flowers to patients for eighteen years, and she was ninety-five!

Two remarkable developments occurred in 1998. Of the 350 to 400 volunteers, more and more males participated—about 25 percent of the total. And so many young people wanted to volunteer that the director of volunteers had to turn some down. Clearly the relationship between Baptist Hospital and the community remains strong.

Chapter 10
MUSIC, SPORTS, AND HEALTH CARE

A big thank you to my friends at Baptist for the wonderful care that my baby and I received during our stay with you. We feel we are very lucky to have such a fine hospital to go to when we need one.
—Barbara Mandrell Dudney

PUBLIC APPEARANCES ARE PART OF THE JOB FOR music celebrities and sports celebrities. Beginning in the mid-1980s, however, their appearances as spokespersons on behalf of Baptist Hospital were unusual. For one thing, hospitals in the Nashville area had only recently begun to advertise their services, and Baptist's administrators had been reluctant to join in that endeavor. For another thing, the celebrities did the work out of respect for the hospital and charged no fees. Some even went so far as to pay for *all* the promotional costs of the advertisements.

For the most part Baptist's administrators had hoped that the whole advertising issue would just go away. Advertising a hospital seemed a bit unprofessional in 1985. Nevertheless, other hospitals had created such a competitive healthcare environment that Baptist Hospital had to get into the advertising flow. But how?

One day David Stringfield brought up the issue to Jerry Reed, singer, guitar player, songwriter, and actor. He admitted that the hospital

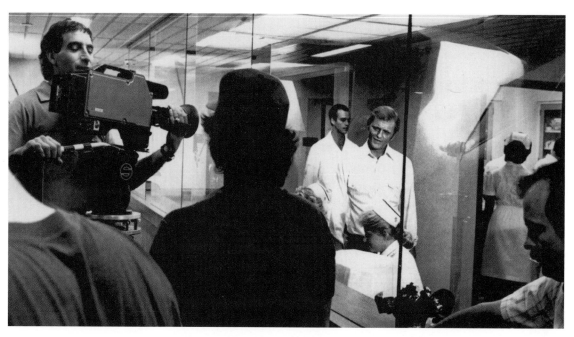

Jerry Reed was the first of many stars to donate their time as spokespersons for Baptist Hospital.

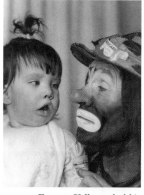

Emmett Kelly worked his clown "magic" on a young patient.

had no experience in such a venture and asked about the best way to begin. Reed volunteered to do the first TV ad, which appeared in May 1985. Reed also encouraged Stringfield to contact other celebrities since Stringfield had become close personal friends with many of them. From having babies to undergoing heart surgery some celebrities had personal experiences in Baptist. Others had friends or family as patients or just wanted to thank the hospital for its good work in the community.

The advertising and marketing program was—and is—a huge success. Debby Patterson Koch has been instrumental in that success. Currently the vice president of communications and marketing, she participated in the production of that first TV ad and over the years has continued to heighten the community's awareness of the hospital through the advertising and marketing program. David Stringfield stated, "As more hospitals began to have advertising and utilize marketing surveys, it was obvious that Baptist Hospital must compete. We could not have found a more dedicated, loyal, and hardworking person than Debby Koch, who had served as Governor Lamar Alexander's press spokesperson. Baptist Hospital has been blessed to have Debby direct these activities and assist in placing Baptist as the number one hospital in all surveys."

Of course, celebrities had been coming to the hospital for various reasons for years. Emmett Kelly visited Baptist in 1968 and 1969 and,

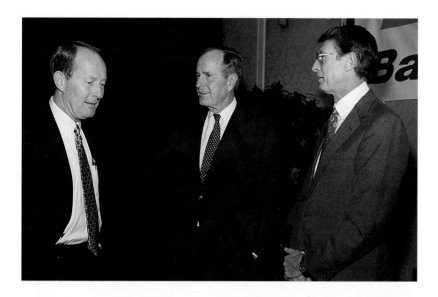

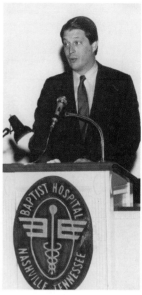

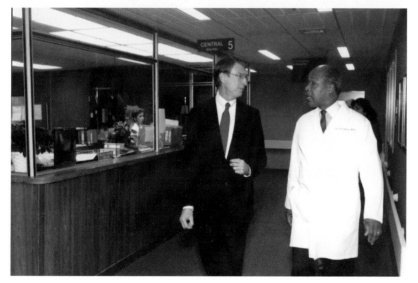

Above left:
Joined by former Governor Lamar Alexander and David Stringfield, former President George Bush was in town to unveil a survey recognizing Baptist Hospital's exceptional results in its heart program.

Above:
When he was a U.S. senator, Al Gore spoke before a Pastor's Conference at Baptist.

Left:
Then Secretary of Health and Human Services Louis Sullivan, M.D., toured the hospital with David Stringfield and commended Baptist's "commitment to a healthy nation" on a visit in 1992.

as his famous clown character, delighted patients, especially in pediatrics and the play room. Elvis Presley's stay in 1971 created a different kind of excitement. Governor Winfield Dunn made it a point to call on him in the hospital.

Garth Brooks, Barbara Mandrell, Wynonna, Waylon Jennings, Alan Jackson, Steve Winwood, Paul Overstreet, Amy Grant, Lionel Cartwright, Lee Greenwood, Suzy Bogguss, Crystal Gayle, Billy Dean, Peter Frampton, and Irlene Mandrell have all had babies born at Baptist.

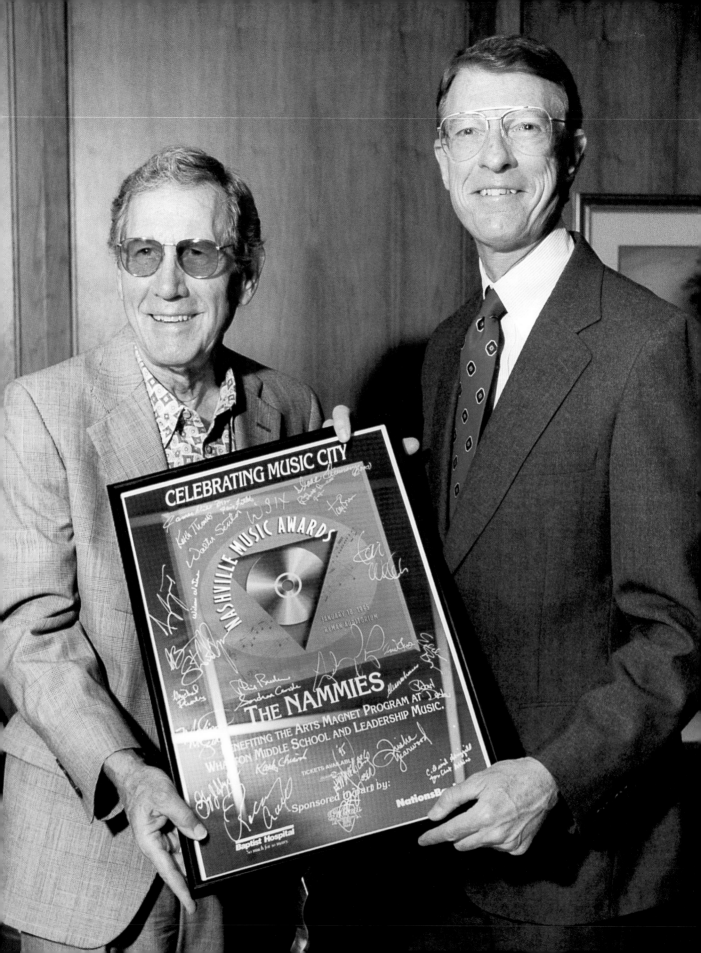

They recognized the hospital's special place in the community when it came to the delivery of babies—more than half of the number of births in the community occur at Baptist.

Following heart bypass surgery in 1989, Waylon Jennings said, "My care at Baptist was wonderful. I couldn't have asked for better treatment." He also mentioned his personal rehabilitation program to monitor his condition. "Since the birth of our son Shooter," he said, "Jessi and I have relied on Baptist." Other performers who have had bypass surgery at Baptist include Johnny Cash, Bill Monroe, George Jones, and Ferlin Husky.

The list of celebrity friends who have donated their time is a long one: Garth Brooks, Chet Atkins, Vince Gill, Alan Jackson, Waylon Jennings, Johnny Cash, George Jones, Jerry Reed, Barbara Mandrell, Louise Mandrell, Irby Mandrell, Irlene Mandrell, Randy Travis, Steve Winwood, Charlie Daniels, Crystal Gayle, Loretta Lynn, Baillie and the Boys, Tom T. Hall, George Lindsey, Billy Dean, Rex Allen Sr., and the late Roy Acuff, Bill Monroe, Jerry Clower, and Tammy Wynette.

The relationship between Baptist Hospital and the Mandrell family has been a very special one that spans more than two decades and three generations. The family moved to Nashville in 1969 and have called it home since that time, with Baptist providing health care for their minor scrapes to their major emergencies. Irby has had three heart surgeries, and his wife, Mary, said, "If it hadn't been for Baptist, we would have lost Irby." They celebrated the births of

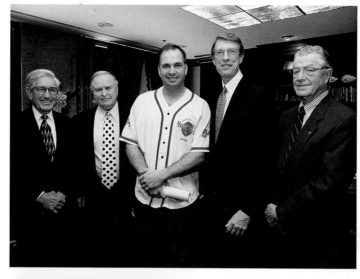

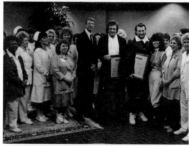

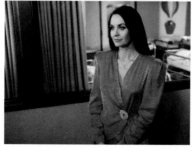

Above:
Garth Brooks met with members of the Baptist Board of Trustees after being one of the hospital's very first patients to undergo a PET (Positron Emission Tomography) scan.
From left to right: Willie Davis, Guy Bates, Garth Brooks, David Stringfield, and Ed Moody.

Center:
Hospital personnel surround David Stringfield, Johnny Cash, Waylon Jennings, and Jessi Colter. Both Cash and Jennings have been patients and spokespersons for the hospital.

Lower left:
Crystal Gale has generously given her time to promote Baptist Hospital's programs and services.

Opposite page:
Chet Atkins and David Stringfield celebrate Music City at a Baptist luncheon honoring the world-famous guitar picker.

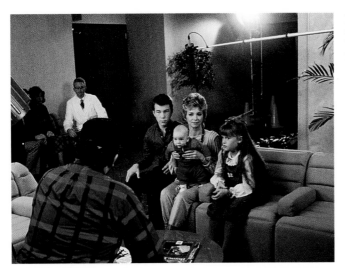

Barbara Mandrell's three children join her for a television announcement about Baptist's care. Barbara spent months at the hospital and in rehabilitation following a car accident in which she was severely injured.

Barbara's and Irlene's children, and Barbara's care and recovery in 1984 from a terrible car accident in which she suffered numerous injuries including a badly damaged right knee, a broken right leg, a concussion, and a fractured ankle. To thank Baptist, the family members have been spokespersons and taped television announcements, and Louise was the driving force behind one of the most successful and spectacular fund-raising banquets in the history of Nashville.

The Mandrell Heart Center was dedicated on November 21, 1996, in recognition of the family's close ties to the hospital. Irby commented, "I have three beautiful daughters but I don't have any sons to carry on the Mandrell name. I feel so honored that Baptist Hospital will carry on the family name long after I'm gone." The Mandrell Heart Center offers a full range of cardiac services, from prevention and community education programs to medical intervention, surgery, and cardiac rehabilitation.

David Stringfield's friendship with a nationally recognized sports figure eventually resulted in a program dedicated to sports medicine and with it came many sports celebrities. Stringfield described the starting point: "Tom Landry, coach of the Dallas Cowboys, was a really good friend. We had become associated through the Fellowship of Christian Athletes. The Cowboys had orthopedic physicians who specialized in sports injuries. Tom encouraged us to have a sports medicine division of orthopaedics since we already had an outstanding orthopedic department. Following Tom's recommendation, I encouraged our orthopedic doctors to have a physician specializing in sports medicine. Over time, we had more and more orthopedic doctors that specialized in just sports medicine to move to Baptist Hospital."

In 1985 Baptist Hospital established a Tom Landry Award given periodically to an individual whose lifestyle stands for what Landry's stands for—keeping spiritually and physically fit. The first recipient was Landry; and due to Stringfield's friendship, others have come to Baptist Hospital to receive the award, such as former Dallas Cowboys quarterback Roger Staubach, former Chicago Bears running back Walter Payton, former Washington Redskins coach Joe Gibbs, former

Chicago Bears coach Mike Ditka, and former Philadelphia 76ers star Julius Erving. Landry said of the 1995 recipient, Olympic gold medal winner Jackie Joyner-Kersee: "Today's athletes are often portrayed in only one dimension—as the athlete, not the complete person. It is important to also show the off-the-field character of these great athletes. [Her] dedication to inner-city kids through her Community Foundation is an excellent illustration of an athlete who believes in giving back to the community that gave her so much." When each of these internationally known athletes received the award, community leaders and youngsters were invited to the ceremony to hear their inspirational remarks.

The late Wilma Rudolph, a world-famous, world-class athlete in her own right, was a vice president on Baptist hospital's administrative staff. She was instrumental in making arrangements for Joyner-Kersee's award. To honor her pledge to Rudolph, Joyner-Kersee came to Nashville to receive the Landry Award and do a television endorsement on behalf of the hospital following Rudolph's untimely death.

Baptist's Sports Medicine program and the Fitness Center share similar goals. Stringfield noted the reasons behind the Baptist Fitness Center, which opened in 1985. "It became apparent that people wanted to know more of what they could do in a preventive way to eliminate any future health problems. We know that eating right, exercising, not being overweight or a cigarette smoker, and trying to eliminate high blood pressure and stress are effective in having a longer, more quality life. All that reduces the risk factors for heart disease and cancer. As people became more interested in disease prevention, the hospital became more involved in educating people. That was when the community education programs began. That was about the time that we built the Fitness Center, which is for the public as well as our employees. I had read that if a person was faithful in exercising three times a week for an hour, absenteeism would be reduced about 50 percent. I was interested in that for Baptist Hospital but also for other corporate leaders and other citizens in general.

"So we started a Fitness Center. Tom Landry and Dr. Ken Cooper of the Aerobics Center in Dallas, Texas, who was a world-famous author of many publications and books and also a friend of Tom Landry and of mine, helped to design the center and recommend certain programs for the center. Dr. Cooper has probably done more throughout the world to promote fitness and a healthy quality of life than anyone. He and Tom Landry are legends in their own time because both believe in keeping spiritually and physically fit." The Baptist Health and Fitness

"I was at Baptist Hospital for outpatient surgery, and would like to express my thanks to the staff. I have always sworn by Baptist Hospital, and when you get such terrific people to work on you in such an overwhelming and sometimes cold, impersonal and terrifying situation, this really counts so much. Thanks so much for your facilities and great employees!"

—Connie Kaylor

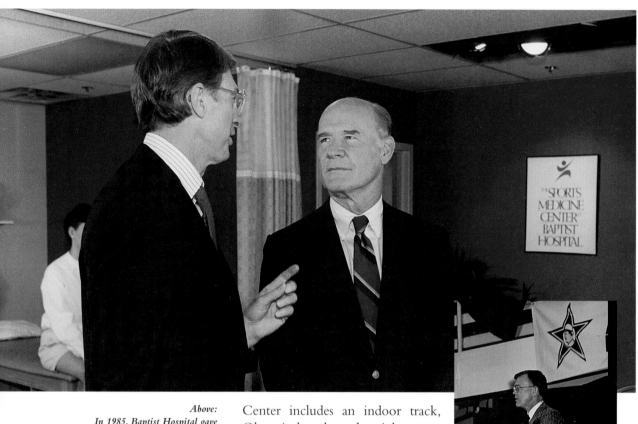

Above:
In 1985, Baptist Hospital gave the first Tom Landry Award to Coach Tom Landry of the Dallas Cowboys. The award honors people who are devoted to keeping spiritually and physically fit.

Inset:
Washington Redskins Coach Joe Gibbs was a recipient of the Landry award in 1988.

Opposite page:
Tom Landry Award Winners Coach Mike Ditka (top left) Walter Payton (bottom center) Julius "Dr. J." Erving (bottom left) Roger Staubach (top right) Olympian Jackie Joyner-Kersee (bottom right).

Center includes an indoor track, Olympic-length pool, weight room, multipurpose gym, steam and sauna rooms, and a therapeutic massage area, and it offers aerobic exercise programs. Dr. Cooper and his wife, Millie, have conducted free seminars on exercise at the center over the years. David Evans, the director of the center at the time it opened, commented, "Of all the fitness centers in the world, Baptist Health and Fitness Center is one of ten for whom Cooper acts as a consultant." In addition to being a facility to exercise, the Health and Fitness Center is used for rehabilitation of orthopedic injuries, cardiac rehabilitation, and other medical-related matters.

When the Baptist Hospital Sports Medicine program began, Ron Bargatze was the director; the current director is Ronn Hollis. Hollis emphasized that the center is for both competitive and recreational athletes. One of only a few in the Southeast, the Sports Medicine program is dedicated to the prevention, care, and treatment of athletic

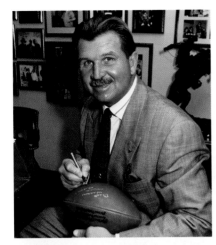

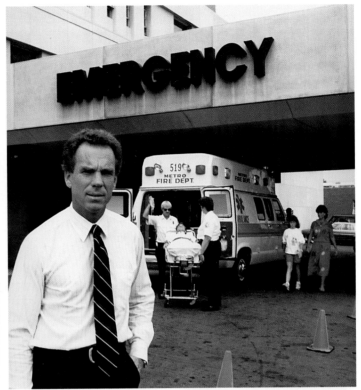

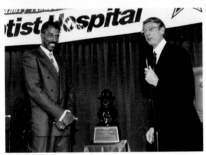

and recreational injuries with the goal of increasing health and assuring a mobile lifestyle in the long term. Through training techniques, diagnostic testing, and evaluation to prevent injuries, the Sports Medicine staff prepare athletes to be able to play a sport and to be able to avoid debilitating problems. Two of the outpatient surgical suites, located below the center, have a closed circuit video

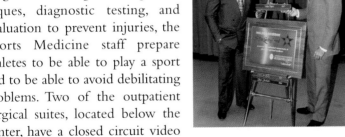

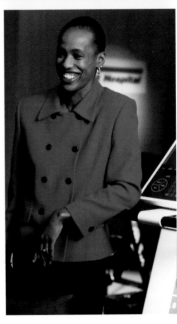

system that enables trainers and physicians to observe and learn from advanced sports medicine surgical techniques.

The center's sports medicine physicians, certified athletic trainers, and therapists have been trainers for the U.S. Sports Festival, World University Games, Pre-Olympic Games, and World Championship Games. And here in the Middle Tennessee area

Baptist sends certified athletic trainers to athletic events held by nineteen high schools and colleges; for example in 1995, they covered several hundred events, which required several thousand hours—all at no charge to the schools. They also train student trainers. The center provides free sports screenings for high school and middle school students. Over the course of the last five years, more than fifteen thousand young athletes have been screened.

The Tennessee Oilers football team announced in 1997 that they had chosen the Baptist Hospital Sports Medicine program as their exclusive healthcare provider. The final decision makers for the selection were owner Bud Adams and team executive Tommy Smith. Head Coach Jeff Fisher said, "The team's decision to select Baptist was based on a number of important factors. In the final analysis, it was Baptist's reputation in the local community, the nature of their involvement in community causes, their outstanding record in the sports medicine field

The Tennessee Oilers selected Baptist Hospital as the team's official healthcare provider. Coach Jeff Fisher and David Stringfield form a strong partnership.

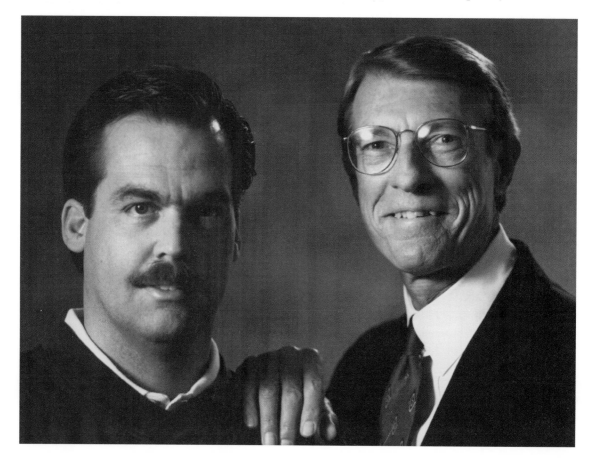

and the opportunities which we mutually embraced." As a unique feature of this partnership, every baby born in 1998 at the hospital goes home with a Tennessee Oilers Future Player Contract, which says, "May this document remind you that with a healthy body and a quick mind, you will be able to tackle anything this new life might throw you. So, stay healthy and go get 'em!" The first baby to receive one was Cameron Christopher Hall, the son of Oiler linebacker LeManski Hall.

Owner Craig Leipold and President Jack Diller of the Nashville Predators hockey team announced in March 1998 that Baptist Hospital would be the NHL team's healthcare provider. In his remarks about the decision Diller said, "While there are several quality healthcare operations in Nashville, we believe Baptist Hospital, with its history in sports medicine, offers us the widest and best range of services to ensure our players are mentally and physically able to compete at the highest level." The medical team includes specialists in orthopaedics, ophthalmology, internal medicine, dentistry, and plastic surgery.

With the Tennessee Golf Association, Baptist Sports Medicine staff members cover the Sara Lee Classic in the spring and The Vinny golf tournament in August. The hospital and the association plan to create some special programs together. The association recognizes that some individuals have unique problems and challenges, perhaps because of physical limitations, but by having a sports medical team observe their swings and make suggestions, the individuals may work toward a better result.

Sports medicine is a relatively new specialty, and its future holds more technology and more noninvasive procedures. Arthroscopic surgery makes rehabilitation easier, and recovery time may be as little as three to six weeks. Scientists now are working toward a needle-size instrument to accomplish the same surgery. In addition synthetic ligaments and reconstituted cartilage are being discussed as real possibilities.

Complementing the Sports Medicine program are the Baptist Orthopedic Center and the Baptist Foot and Ankle Center. The Orthopedic Center staff treats musculoskeletal disorders, broken bones, torn ligaments, and dislocations, and offers rehabilitation

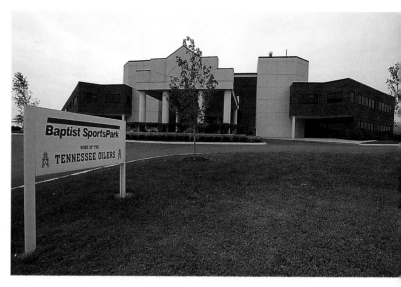

Baptist Hospital Sports Park

"Just a quick note to compliment Baptist Hospital for providing free ColoCare kits to the public. This clearly reflects the emphasis Baptist puts on preventive health care and the quality of that decision. Thank you."

—Kay Bjork

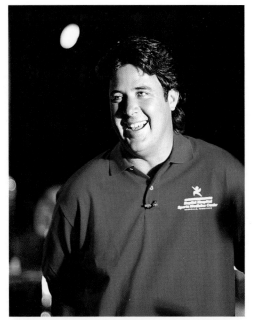

services. The professionals at the Foot and Ankle Center can care for conditions from bunions to unexplained pain in feet and ankles; there are also educational programs for good foot health.

The Right Team, a partnership between Baptist Sports Medicine and the Tennessee Secondary School Athletic Association, encourages abstinence from drugs, alcohol, and tobacco while stressing physical fitness to middle and high school students. The objective of the Right Team is to help students make the "right" choice about these substances. On their off days, Oilers players accompany the Right Team staffers to Middle Tennessee schools, and plans are under way to involve the Predators too. Many schools across the state have requested a Right Team program.

These sports celebrities have joined the music celebrities in donating their time on behalf of Baptist Hospital to do advertisements: race car driver Darrell Waltrip, Coach Tom Landry, Coach Mike Ditka, basketball player Julius Erving, quarterback Roger Staubach, Coach Joe Gibbs, the Washington Redskins team, running back Walter Payton, track star Jackie Joyner-Kersee, Dr. Ken Cooper and his wife, Millie Cooper, quarterback Danny White, defensive lineman Randy White, football great Bill Bates, running back Herschel Walker, defensive lineman Ed "Too Tall" Jones,

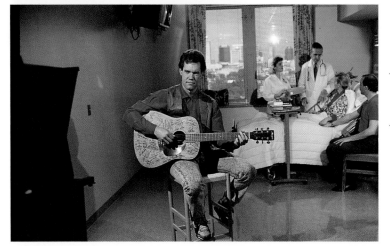

Superstar entertainers Vince Gill (top) and Randy Travis (above) have both been incredibly supportive of Baptist, not only by filming commercials, but in supporting the Foundation.

football player Doug Cosbie, Coach Ken Dugan, and Coach Jeff Fisher. Baptist Hospital is grateful for their contributions and for their confidence in the hospital and its services.

Chapter 11

A LOOK AHEAD

It's a Christian institution for healing.
—Guy E. Bates Sr.
Chairman, Board of Trustees

FROM AN INDIAN VILLAGE ON THE BANKS OF THE Cumberland River to a tiny settlement of white pioneers to a major American city, Nashville has come a long way. Now, in 1998, ranked as the twenty-first largest metropolitan area in the nation, Nashville has earned the position of one of the top healthcare centers in the United States, perhaps the world, a distinction that draws as much attention to the city as the Grand Ole Opry.

How could that happen in a relaxed southern city, more famous for country music and religious publishing than for the often overlooked quality of its medical facilities? There were many factors: the reputation of Vanderbilt University Medical Center as a research and teaching facility; the progressive leadership of other local hospitals, led by Baptist Hospital; and the advent of the for-profit chains founded by a former Baptist board chairman and others. Today, hundreds of separate Nashville-based companies are engaged in some aspect of healthcare delivery, and many other support firms are clustered around the corporate healthcare complex.

Before gazing into the future of health care in Nashville, we need to examine the roots, the reasons, and the chronology of this phenomenon. Protestant Hospital was founded in 1918, born of a devastating flu epidemic that convinced local leaders that more healthcare facilities were vital to the life of the city. Over time, the hospital fell deeply into debt and would not have survived without thoughtful and courageous intervention. It became Mid-State Baptist Hospital in 1948, and

117

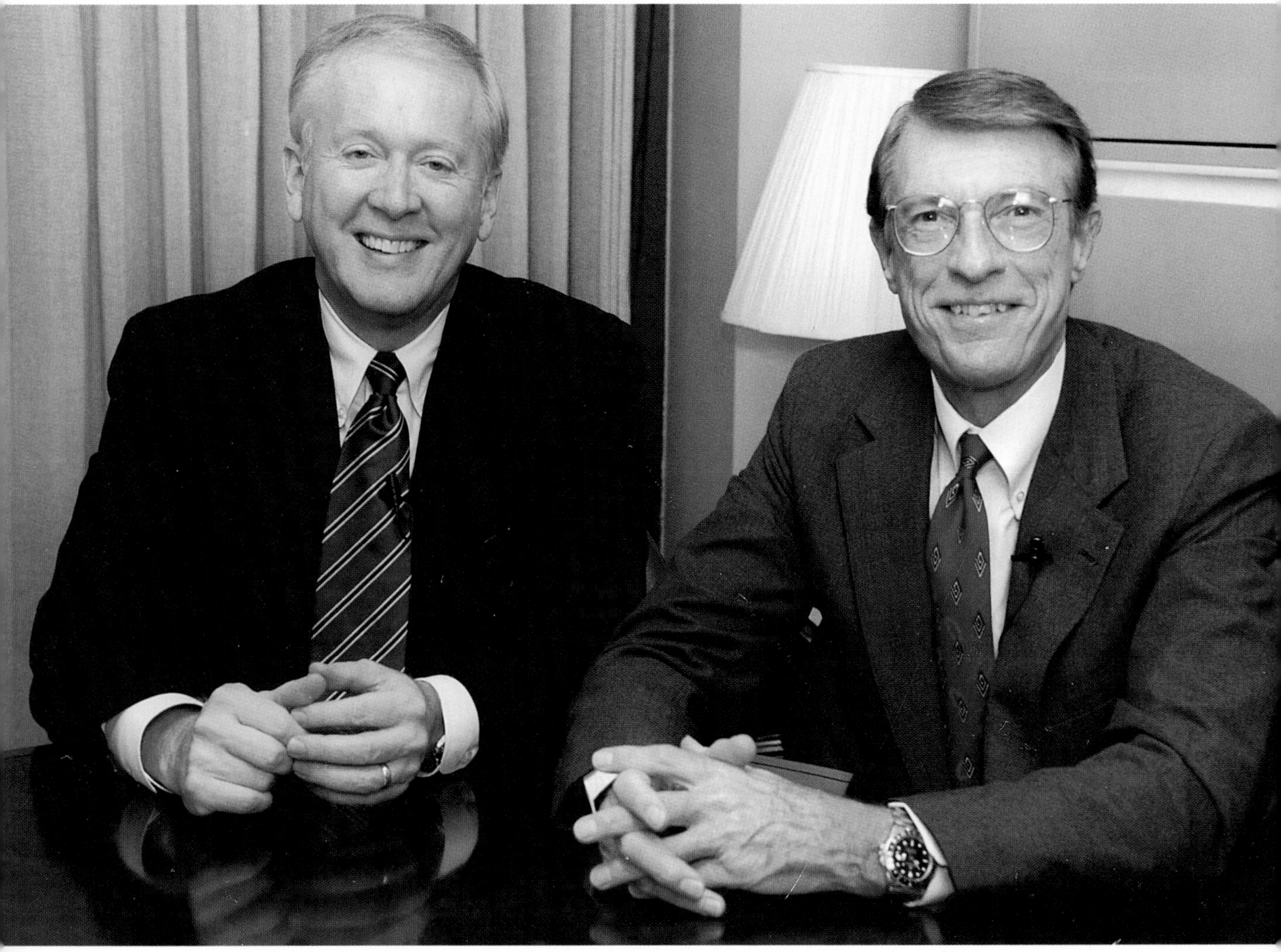

Effective October 1, 1998, Erie Chapman became the new president and CEO of Baptist Hospital, and David Stringfield became chairman of the Board of Trustees.

in 1964 simply Baptist Hospital. Early progress was slow; the dramatic growth was to come much later.

As David Stringfield said in the summer of 1998, "Gene Kidd's leadership and the leadership of the board, and the improvements that they made in the physicians that they recruited, turned the hospital around from a money-losing proposition. Gene Kidd and the board built a great foundation that we have been able to build on."

The Rev. Dr. Franklin Paschall, a former board chairman, added details to Mr. Stringfield's statement: "In my term we moved from a kind of clinic, a somewhat small operation, to building buildings and into an era of high-tech medicine. We had to make a decision—and I was part of that—to have an updated hospital in terms of equipment, as good as could be found anywhere. I consider the updated equipment, not just the buildings, in Baptist Hospital very important in the history of its growth and development and service.

"You can ruin a hospital in a short time," Paschall continued, "when the word goes out that these people are behind. We want to be a hospital where people can be referred from these small towns for the best medicine. . . . Hospitals that stay in the top echelon—that means money. And obviously it takes money to grow a hospital, to keep pace with advancing technology, and to provide the services the community needs."

"The real era of growth started in 1982, when David Stringfield was promoted to the position of president and CEO of Baptist," stated Guy Bates. With the full backing of a progressive Board of Trustees, a quality medical staff, and dedicated employees and administrative staff members, he launched an expansion and improvement campaign that by 1998 had totaled nearly $500 million in new investments in the facility. More than one hundred new programs began in addition to the building program.

Concurrently, the first of the for-profit chains were gaining momentum in Nashville and spreading their brand of health care across the nation. The two opposing forces, Nashville's largest six not-for-profit hospitals and the for-profit chains, were actually somewhat synergistic in bringing growth and progress to the healthcare industry. All prospered.

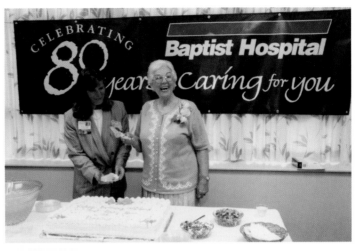

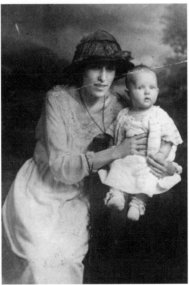

Above:
In March 1998, Baptist Hospital hosted a birthday party at the Women's Pavilion for the hospital's first patient, Anita Kilby Lewis. She was born on March 20, 1919.

Left:
Gladys Kilby holds her young daughter, Anita.

*The hospital awarded a certificate
to the one millionth patient,
Marvin G. Thomasson, in 1976.*

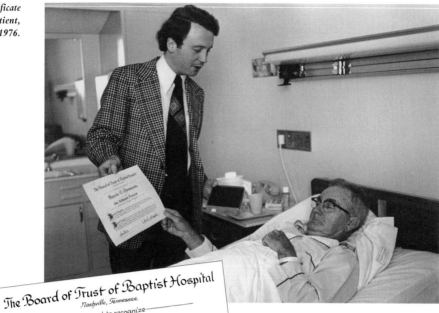

Both groups met the new challenges of the 1980s and 1990s, with increasing government involvement in health care, skyrocketing healthcare costs, the onset of managed care in its various forms, and the closer bonding of hospitals with the physicians who admit patients.

It was a time of massive change in the healthcare industry.

"Some of the most difficult obstacles in the past," Stringfield explained, "were to keep pace in a competitive market with what other hospitals and healthcare institutions were doing. At that time we had to work extremely hard to keep pace and to get ahead of what other hospitals were doing. We have been blessed with a great team of board members, physicians, employees, and administrative staff."

It was also a time to look to the future and make plans.

Modern technology and an array of new medical procedures had continually made hospital stays shorter and shifted emphasis from acute care to preventive medicine and outpatient surgery and other treatment. Large inpatient hospitals would always be important, but there was no longer room for growth in acute care beds.

The emphasis had to be on utilizing the new methods to meet the needs of the consuming public, taking health care into the suburbs and small towns surrounding Nashville, forming alliances with physicians to assure an adequate market share, taking advantage of every practical new development in technology and medical advances, and seizing new innovations in maintaining a healthy population in the area served by the hospital.

Stringfield said, "Healthcare advances have made it possible for people to live even longer. That is one of the reasons healthcare costs are going up. It has been projected by the federal government that as much as 50 percent of the Medicare budget is spent on patients whose bills are incurred during the last week of their lives. That is a significant statistic.

"Each new program means additional equipment and additional highly trained personnel and that all adds to the costs," Stringfield continued. "Seventy-five percent of what we have in our pharmacy was not available even ten years ago. It would be unconscionable for a hospital not to have these new drugs, but they are costly to develop and costly to stock. This is just one example of what I mean by the costs and the challenges we have in meeting consumers' needs."

The two millionth patient was Laura Brinton, daughter of Lisa and Larry Brinton Jr., who arrived in 1988. Dr. H. Franklin Paschall, then chairman of the board, and David Stringfield presented gifts to Mrs. Brinton.

Stringfield stressed, "Baptist Hospital is a Christian hospital. That's first and foremost, and as a Christian hospital, there needs to be a demonstration of greater love, greater empathy, greater sympathy. We are blessed with a wonderful chaplain's program that ministers to spiritual needs of patients. We feel that a well-rounded program for patients ministers not only to their physical needs but their spiritual and emotional needs as well."

Looking to the future, Stringfield remarked, "Saving money for patients and having easy access will drive health care in the future. Physicians and hospitals must concentrate on both.

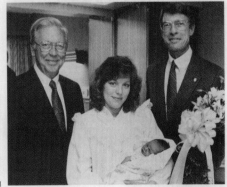

BAPTIST ADMITS TWO MILLIONTH PATIENT

Lisa Brinton was honored as the two millionth patient to be admitted to Baptist Hospital. Mrs. Brinton delivered Laura Michelle, a 7 pound, 9½ ounce baby girl. It is the second child for her and her husband, Larry Brinton, Jr., who is employed in the Court Clerk's office of Metropolitan Government.

Baptist Hospital traces its beginning to the year 1918 and the old Protestant Hospital. Ownership of the hospital was transferred to the Tennessee Baptist Convention in April 1948. It has grown from 200 beds to its present 750-bed capacity.

C. David Stringfield, president, noted that the first patient admitted to Baptist on March 20, 1919, was a maternity patient who delivered a baby girl. "We admitted our one millionth patient 57 years later," he added, "a cardiac patient from Alabama in May 1976. Indicative of our growth is the fact that just 12 years later, we have admitted our two millionth patient.

"Baptist Hospital has built its reputation for quality care on a solid foundation of concern and professionalism," Stringfield said, "combined with the most comprehensive, state-of-the-art medical technology available. We look forward to treating our next two million patients in the same manner."

A special package of services was presented to Mrs. Brinton, including two round trip tickets to anywhere in the continental U.S. on American Airlines, courtesy of Travel Time, Inc. To help ease the transition into motherhood, she also received eight hours of "Mother's Helper" home care services from Baptist Hospital Home Care and free enrollment in

Dr. H. Franklin Paschall, chairman of the board, and Mr. C. David Stringfield, present Mrs. Larry Brinton with a special package of gifts.

Working Parents and Especially Grandparents classes at the Baptist Women's Pavilion.

Mrs. Brinton also received two free memberships at the Baptist Health & Fitness Center and enrollment in Shapes Unique post-partum exercise class at Baptist.

"Here are some specifics. More and more procedures are going to be done on an outpatient basis. In our busy culture easy access will become more important and more available with walk-in clinics. More advances in medicine will be made. Not that long ago patients who had gallbladder surgery were in the hospital for a week or ten days, but now a stay of twenty-four to forty-eight hours is more typical. Similar illustrations apply to hip replacement and many other surgical procedures. Pharmacy costs will continue to rise as exciting new medicines become available. More specialized procedures will be done in communities outside major cities because the communities want this and medical schools are training more and more specialists. Some states have a surplus of specialists. Those people are going to go where they can find work. More home care will occur. The baby boomers won't overload hospitals because of the trend toward outpatient treatment. A surplus of hospital beds is imminent, which means less traditional hospital buildings but more outpatient facilities."

Stringfield observed, "Most patients will be involved in one managed care plan or another, with their continuum of care prescribed by their insurance carrier or other third-party payer. This will result in an increasing number of conflicts between healthcare providers, physicians, and payers over the type, quantity, and cost of treatment allowed for the individual patient. The issue of 'the right to care' will become increasingly significant."

"How would you feel, sitting in a doctor's office, being told that you had a tumor underneath your brain affecting your sight.? During the three months following the tumor surgery at Baptist Hospital I had twenty-five radiation treatments. For an old retired colonel, my golf game sure did improve."

—*Col. John Hill, retired*

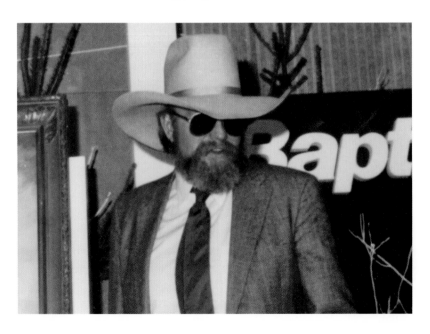

Charlie Daniels is another celebrity who has been supportive of Baptist Hospital. He has taped, at his own expense, two television spots promoting Baptist's care and services.

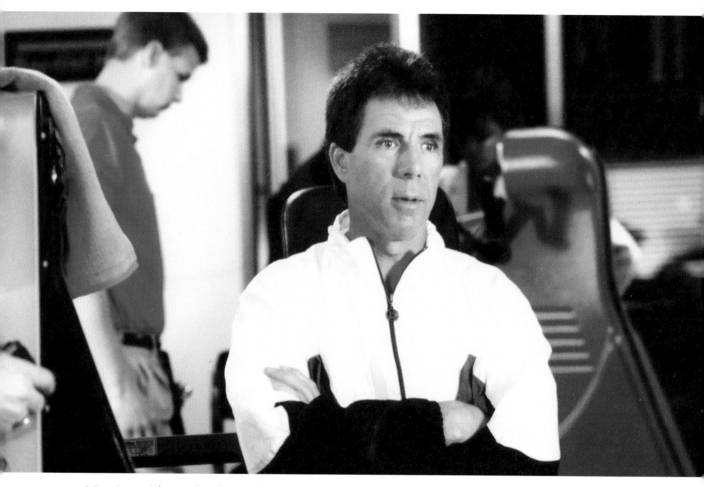

Merging with another hospital had been considered as a way to better serve the community, contain costs, and strengthen the leadership of the not-for-profit sector. Preliminary talks had been conducted with Vanderbilt University Medical Center. Extensive work was done with Saint Thomas Hospital over the period of a year, but negotiations with Saint Thomas were called off in May 1998, with the following public statement: "We have concluded that each institution can accomplish its mission and serve the needs of our patients and employees and the community by looking for specific ways to work together rather than merging operations at this time." Both institutions agreed that such conversations might be resumed at some point in the future.

In July 1998, at the age of fifty-nine and after thirty years of service at Baptist Hospital, Stringfield recommended a plan of transition and

Race car driver Darrell Waltrip crashed at the Daytona 500 and spent many months in rehabilitation at Baptist. On a happier note, he and his wife, Stevie, had their children at Baptist as well.

succession for the position of president/CEO and assisted the Board of Trustees in selecting his successor as president and CEO, and he accepted a promotion to the position of board chairman. At that time, too, Virgil Moore was named chairman of the Executive Committee. The new head of the hospital, a nationally recognized hospital management specialist, took office October 1, 1998. He is Erie Chapman, a fifty-four-year-old attorney who had been president and CEO of large healthcare systems in Ohio and Florida, and consulted with a number of other healthcare organizations.

Both men talked of "teamwork" in managing the future direction of Baptist Hospital, with Stringfield assuming responsibility for long-range planning, direction of future mergers, acquisitions, other new

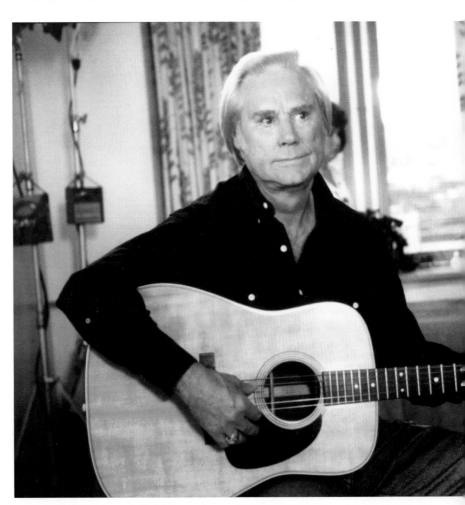

The enduring quality of George Jones's music has guaranteed him an esteemed place in the country music world, and his relationship with Baptist Hospital has had a similar enduring quality.

relationships, and fund-raising, while Chapman assumed control of daily operations of the entire Baptist system. Stringfield stated, "Erie Chapman is a very capable Christian leader who will be a great director."

On the question of what the future holds, Stringfield said in closing, "We may not know what the future holds, but I think the Lord knows the future and I know that He can guide us in our deliberations and our decisions. There is a great Bible quote that states you should 'trust in the LORD with all your heart, and do not lean on your own understanding. In all your ways acknowledge Him, and He will make your paths straight' (Proverbs 3:5–6), and another that states, 'Seek first His kingdom and His righteousness; and all these things [your daily needs] shall be added to you' (Matthew 6:33)."

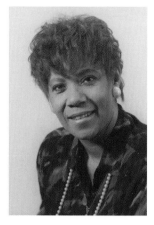

The late Wilma Rudolph, a record-breaking Olympian and Tennessee native, was on the hospital's administrative staff.

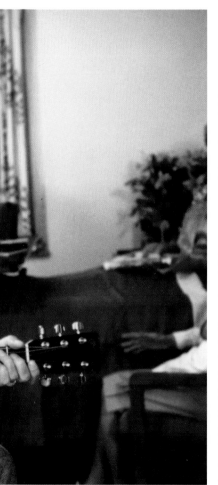

The first patient at Protestant Hospital in 1919 was a baby, Anita Kilby. Fifty-seven years would pass before the one millionth patient, Marvin G. Thomasson, would enter Baptist Hospital in 1976 to receive cardiac care. But it took only twelve more years before the arrival of the two millionth patient, baby Laura Michelle Brinton, in 1988. Given the current medical trends, projecting the entrance of the three millionth patient is difficult. But Baptist Hospital will be prepared to care for him or her, whenever it happens.

Addie Hamilton regularly visits patients in the hospital and always asks two questions: "How are you today? And are we taking good care of you?" Ninety-nine percent give excellent reports on personnel and what they think is happening at Baptist Hospital. Throughout its eighty years, the hospital has had a heritage of healing. Baptist's leadership team has earned a national reputation for advanced thinking, planning, and positive initiatives in meeting tomorrow's healthcare needs today. That commitment will continue into the next century.

Appendix 1
BOARD MEMBERS

**Chairmen of the Board of Trustees
of Baptist Hospital—1948–98**

Jack C. Massey (1948–60)

Charles E. Creagh (1961–63, 1973)

Russell W. Brothers (1964)

A. E. Batts (1965–67)

Lem B. Stevens (1968-72, 1974–76)

James H. Winters (1977–81)

H. Franklin Paschall (1982–88)

Guy E. Bates (1989–98)

C. David Stringfield (1998–)

**Chairman of the Executive Committee
of Baptist Hospital—1998**

Virgil H. Moore Jr. (1998–)

Members of the Board of Trustees of Baptist Hospital—1948–98

Members of the Baptist Health Care System, Inc. Board—1991–98
Board of Trust

MEDICAL STAFF MEMBERS

Chiefs of Staff

1948–54	Charles C. Trabue, M.D.
1954–56	Carl. S. McMurray, M.D.
1956–58	Robert M. Finks, M.D.
1958–61	George K. Carpenter, M.D.
1961–63	Robert L. McCracken, M.D.
1963–65	James N. Thomasson, M.D.
1965–67	James A. Kirtley Jr., M.D.
1967–69	S. Benjamin Fowler, M.D.
1969–71	John M. Tudor, M.D.
1971–73	Russell Birmingham, M.D.
1973–75	R. A. Greer Ricketson, M.D.
1976–77	John L. Farringer Jr., M.D.
1978–79	Douglas H. Riddell, M.D.
1980–81	T. Guv Pennington, M.D.
1982–83	Arthur G. Bond, M.D.
1984–85	William Crenshaw, M.D.
1986–87	Charles E. Mayes, M.D.
1988–89	H. Newt Lovvorn Jr., M.D.
1990–91	John G. Thompson Jr., M.D.
1992–93	Robert A. Hardin, M.D.
1994–95	Ronald E. Overfield, M.D.
1996–97	Edmond F. Tipton, M.D.
1998–99	Eugene M. Regen Jr., M.D.

Medical Staff Officers

Presidents

1946	J. Sumpter Anderson, M.D.
1947–48	Dr. W. J. Core
1949	Harrison H. Shoulders, M.D.
1950	George K. Carpenter, M.D.
1951	Ray O. Fessey, M.D.
1952	James P. Anderson, M.D.
1953	John S. Cayce, M.D.
1954	Elkin L. Rippy, M.D.
1955	Robert M. Finks, M.D.
1956	D. Scott Bayer, M.D.
1957	Robert K. Galloway, M.D.
1957 (July)	James N. Thomasson, M.D.
1958	Joseph McKelvie, M.D.
1959	C. C. Woodcock, M.D.
1960	Douglas H. Riddell, M.D.
1961	S. Benjamin Fowler, M.D.
1962	James N. Thomasson, M.D.
1963	Frank C. Womack, M.D.
1964	James W. Ellis, M.D.
1965	John M. Tudor, M.D.
1966	Joe M. Strayhorn, M.D.
1967	D. Scott Bayer, M.D.
1968	W. Andrew Dale, M.D.
1969	George Holcomb, M.D.
1970	Fred D. Ownby, M.D.
1971	John J. Farringer Jr., M.D.
1972	Charles Hamilton, M.D.
1973	Walter L. Diveley, M.D.
1974	Roy Parker, M.D.
1975	Jackson Harris, M.D.
1976	David Pickens Jr., M.D.
1977	T. Guv Pennington, M.D.
1978	Arthur Bond, M.D.
1979	Horace Lavely Jr., M.D.
1980	John Tanner, M.D.
1981	Ronald Overfield, M.D.
1982	Thomas Parrish, M.D.
1983	George K. Carpenter Jr., M.D.
1984	James W. Hays, M.D.
1985	Robert Hardin, M.D.
1986	H. Newton Lovvorn, M.D.
1987	Richard Oldham, M.D.
1988	Phillip P. Porch Jr., M.D.
1989	Reuben A. Bueno, M.D.
1990	N. Don Hasty, M.D.
1991	Frank E. Jones, M.D.
1992–93	Taylor M. Wray, M.D.
1994–95	James R. Cato, M.D.
1996–97	Michael B. Bottomy, M.D.
1998–99	Keith W. Hagan, M.D.

Secretary-Treasurers

1961–62	J. L. Farringer, M.D.
1963	Fred Cowden, M.D.
1964–65	Charles Hamilton, M.D.
1966–67	James Phythyon, M.D.
1968–69	Richard Ownbey, M.D.
1970–71	Harold Dennison, M.D.
1972	T. Guv Pennington, M.D.
1973	Jackson Harris, M.D.
1974–75	Arthur Bond, M.D.
1976	Irving Hillard, M.D.
1977	Sumpter Anderson Jr., M.D.
1978–79	Ronald Overfield, M.D.
1980–81	Con Potanin, M.D.
1982	Walter Brown, M.D.
1983	Reuben A. Bueno, M.D.
1984	Robert T. Barnett, M.D.
1985	Warren McPherson, M.D.
1986	Robert E. Stein, M.D.
1987	Daryl L. Nichols, M.D.
1988	Robert C. Dunkerley Jr., M.D.
1989	Radford C. Stewart, M.D.
1990	Douglas P. Mitchell, M.D.
1991	John E. Keyser III, M.D.
1992–93	William J. Anderson, M.D.
1994	Tom E. Nesbitt Jr., M.D.
1995–96	Royce T. (Terry) Adkins, M.D.
1997–98	Webb J. Earthman, M.D.

Chiefs of Service, from 1977 to 1998

Anesthesiology
Nelson E. Shankle
Jonathan M. Schwartz
James L. Vincent
John C. Dalton
Thomas F. Shultz

Emergency Medicine
John E. Peters,
William R. Huffman
Norman D. Hasty
David G. Lee
Robert M. Hutton
Mary J. Brown
Robert W. Robinson

Family Practice
George Perler
C. Wesley Emfinger
Gita Mishra

Internal Medicine
Charles E. Mayes
John R. Schweikert
John G. Thompson Jr.
E. B. Anderson
Edmond F. Tipton
Taylor M. Wray
Francis W. Gluck Jr.

Medical Imaging
Ronald E. Overfield
John M. Tanner
Michael B. Seshul

Neuroscience
Harold P. Smith
Richard S. Lisella
Carl R. Hampf

Obstetrics/Gynecology
Harry Baer
B. K. Hibbitt
H. Newton Lovvorn
Norman Witthauer
Charles M. Gill
Frederick L. Finke
H. Clay Newsome III
Carl W. Zimmerman

Ophthalmology
L. Rowe Driver
Terry M. Burkhalter
Spencer P. Thornton
Robert L. Estes
James W. Felch
Ronald E. McFarland
Ralph E. Wesley

Orthopaedics
Frank Jones
Eugene M. Regen Jr.
Mark Doyne
Robert E. Stein
William M. Gavigan
David S. Jones
Mark R. Christofersen

Otolaryngology
Jerrell P. Crook
C. Gary Jackson
John D. Witherspoon
William L. Downey
Ronald C. Cate
Jerrell P. Crook Jr.

Pathology
Frank Womack
Richard R. Oldham

Pediatrics
Arville Wheeler
Harvey Spark
James S. Price
Charles Hirshberg
Joseph F. Lentz
David D. Thombs
Mary Catherine Dundon
Ralph M. Greenbaum

Psychiatry
William Sheridan
Stephen C. Humble

Surgery
John Wright
Harold Dennison
Robert A. Hardin
Terry R. Allen
W. Tyree Finch

Plastic Surgery
R. A. Greer Ricketson
Perry F. Harris

Urology
William B. Crenshaw
Robert T. Barnett
Keith W. Hagan
Robert A. Sewell
John W. Brock III
Charles W. Eckstein
Thomas E. Nesbitt Jr.

Appendix 3
ADMINISTRATORS

The administrative staff from 1954 to 1998.

John Eugene Kidd
    Executive Director
    President
    President Emeritus
C. David Stringfield
    Administrative Director
    Executive Vice President
    President/CEO
    Chairman of the Board
Erie Chapman
    President/CEO
Lawrence E. Acker
    Assistant Vice President,
    General Services
    Vice President,
    Professional Services
William J. Akers
    Senior Vice President,
    Corporate Finance
Jamie L. Amaral
    Vice President,
    Physician Services
Donald L. Bailey
    Vice President,
    Corporate Communications
Fred L. Bell
    Chaplain, Director of
    Religion and Personnel
George U. Bennett
    Executive Vice President,
    Development

John G. Blackman
    Construction
    Coordinator/Engineer
Barbara Brennan
    Associate Vice President
    Vice President, Nursing
Robert P. Brueck
    Assistant Administrator,
    Administrative President
Gary A. Brukardt
    Executive Vice President,
    Healthcare Affiliates
Carey Burke
    Vice President, Operations
John L. Cail
    Vice President, Planning
Lucius W. Carroll, II
    Senior Vice President,
    External Affairs and Development
Clarence G. Cawood
    Director,
    Public Relations
John Chapman
    President, Health Net
James R. Childers
    Vice President,
    Fiscal Affairs
Michael E. Crews
    Vice President and
    Senior Vice President,
    Finance

Susan L. Crutchfield
   Vice President
   Senior Vice President,
   Healthcare Affiliates;
   Vice President,
   Patient Care Services

William C. Day
   Director, Pastoral Services;
   Associate Vice President,
   Counseling,
   Pastoral Services

Mark A. Doyne, M.D.
   Senior Vice President,
   Corporate Development

Nora Durham
   Assistant Vice President,
   Personnel

Betsy B. Edwards
   Legal Counsel

David J. Farmer
   Director, Pastoral Services

James E. Farris, Ph.D.
   Vice President,
   Medical Education

Ray O. Fessey
   Director, Employee Health
   Service

Kim Fetterman
   Vice President, Finance,
   Baptist Properties

William H. Flanagan Jr.
   Vice President, Administration

Timothy Flesch
   Senior Vice President,
   Corporate Finance

William O. Floyd
   Chief Engineer

Samuel B. Fowler III
   Vice President, Operations,
   Baptist Properties;
   Vice President, Administration

Anne C. Franklin
   Director, Public Relations

Francis W. Gluck Jr., M.D.
   Director,
   Ambulatory Medicine;
   Medical Director,
   Fitness Center

James L. Goodloe
   Vice President

Ralph Greene
   Building Manager, MSMC

Luke Gregory
   Senior Vice President,
   Operations

Addie E. Hamilton
   Vice President,
   PM Administrator

Joe Hampton
   Assistant Vice President

Robert A. Hardin, M.D.,
   Director, Medical Affairs

Gerald Hemmer
   Project Engineer;
   Construction Engineer

Terry Hiers Jr.
   Assistant Administrator

Clarence M. Holt
   Administrative Engineer

Michael D. Huggins
   Vice President, Operations

Maxine S. Ingram
   Assistant Vice President,
   Environmental Services;
   Assistant Vice President,
   General Services;
   Assistant Vice President,
   Housekeeping

Robert E. Johnson
   Vice President,
   Communications,
   Marketing, Public Relations

William Johnson
   Supervisor/Director, Nurses;
   Senior Vice President,
   Professional Affairs

James H. Jones III
   Senior Vice President,
   Operations

Aileen Katcher
   Director, Marketing

Jack D. Kennedy
   Director, Marketing

Joanne B. Knight
   Vice President, Home Health;
   Vice President,
   Healthcare Affiliates

Debby Patterson Koch
   Director, Communications;
   Vice President,
   Communications and
   Marketing

Kevin T. Korner
   Vice President,
   Human Resources

Lewis M. Lamberth Jr.
   Director,
   Pastoral Services

Brian A. Lapps
   Executive Director,
   Health Net;
   Senior Vice President,
   Planning and Development

Larry M. Levinson
   Assistant Vice President,
   Vice President

Sue Longcore
   Assistant Vice President,
   Vice President,
   Patient Care Services

Iry E. Lowrey Jr.
   Senior Vice President,
   Fiscal Affairs

Calvin R. MacKay
    Senior Vice President, Executive Vice President,
    Corporate Finance
David M. Maloney
    Vice President, Managed Care
Mark M. Manion
    Chief Engineer
David L. Manning
    Senior Vice President, Professional Services
T. W. Manning
    Director of Parking, Administrative Assistant
William C. Mays
    Hospital Chaplain, Director,
    Pastoral Services, Education
Paul C. McNabb II, M.D.
    Medical Director,
    Internal Medicine Residency Program
Lawrence V. Meagher
    Executive Vice President, Baptist Properties
James H. Miller
    Assistant Administrator, Professional Services
John D. Miller
    Vice President, Healthcare Affiliates
Paul W. Moore
    Vice President, Public Relations;
    Senior Vice President,
    Executive Vice President
Wilma S. Newton
    Vice President, Finance
John T. Olive
    Operations Manager, Assistant Vice President
Martha B. Olsen
    Vice President, Human Resources
James W. Palmer
    Controller, Assistant Administrator,
    Business Affairs
Richard Panek
    Vice President, Clinic Operations
Jack L. Parish
    Assistant Vice President,
    Professional Affairs

Laura Pitts
    Director, Community Relations
David A. Purcell
    Vice President, Finance
Robert E. Rippy
    Vice President, Materials Management
Virginia Robertson
    Assistant Vice President, Personnel
Edward A. Rogers Jr., M.D.
    Director, Medical Education
Lawrence E. Ross
    Assistant Administrator,
    Purchasing and Building Services; Vice President
Wilma Rudolph
    Vice President
Glen Sesler
    Director, Vice President, Purchasing
Robert N. Sherrod Sr.
    Assistant Administrator, Senior Vice President
Barry M. Spero
    Assistant Administrator, Administrative Director
Evelyn S. Springer
    Vice President, Nursing Service;
    Senior Vice President, Patient Care Services
Janie F. Sullivan
    Director, Nursing
James B. Swearingen
    Vice President, Finance
Jim Thompson
    Administrative Assistant
Mel Thompson
    Assistant Vice President
Thomas J. Troy
    Executive Vice President, Affiliates
John Tudor, M.D.
    Director, Medical Affairs
Arthur D. Victorine
    Senior Vice President, External Affairs
W. T. Victory Jr.
    Vice President, Personnel,
    Corporate Health Services

Larry D. Walker
    Vice President, Healthcare Affiliates
Cameron Welton
    Vice President, Senior Vice President, Operations
Rachel M. West
    Assistant Vice President, Human Resources
Steve West
    Vice President, Marketing
O. Michael Williams
    Administrative Assistant
Walter H. Williams
    Assistant Administrator
James E. Word
    Senior Vice President, Healthcare Affiliates
Charles E. Yancey
    Vice President, Risk Management;
    Vice President, Administration

Appendix 4
CORPORATE ADVISORY BOARD

Bob Arnett, Vice President and General Manager
    Toshiba America Consumer Products, Inc.
Jim Beard, President
    Caterpillar Financial
Jerry Benefield, President
    Nissan Motor Manufacturing Corporation
Ed Benson Jr., Executive Director
    Country Music Association
Denny Bottorff, Chairman and CEO
    First American Corporation
James C. Bradford Jr., Senior Partner
    J. C. Bradford and Company
Tony Brown, President
    MCA Records
W. Michael Clevy
    International Comfort Products Corporation
Matthew C. Cordaro, President and CEO
    Nashville Electric Service
Gary B. Crigger, Senior Vice President Business Planning
    Bridgestone/Firestone, Inc.
Mike Curb, President
    Curb Records
Brownlee Currey
    Currey Investments
Bill Denny
    Denny Properties
Frank DeTillio, Vice President and General Manager
    WSMV-TV
Tim DuBois, President
    Arista Records
DeWitt Ezell, President
    BellSouth

R. Walter Hale III, Executive Vice President
Trust and Investment Management for Tennessee
Sun Trust Bank

Donna Hilley, President and CEO
Sony/ATV Tree

Joe Hudson (Retired)
(Ford Motor Glass Plant)

Burt Hummell (Retired)
(Robert Orr Sysco)

Doug Hutchins, Division Vice President
Whirlpool Corporation

Clyde F. Ingalls, Regional Vice President
First Tennessee Bank

Orrin Ingram, Copresident
Ingram Industries

Lillian B. Jenkins, Vice President Human Resources
Aladdin Industries

Lem Lewis, General Manager
WTVF

Thomas McCarthy, Plant Manager
DuPont

Allen A. McCampbell Jr., Vice President and
Assistant to President
American General Life and Accident Insurance

Deb McDermott, Vice President and General Manager
WKRN

Craig Moon, Publisher and President
The Tennessean

Kitty Moon, President
Scene Three

Ed Overbey, President
Castner Knott

Dave Reiland, CFO and Executive Vice President
MagneTek

David Roddey, Executive Vice President
NationsBank

Pat Rolfe, Director of Member Relations
ASCAP

John Terzo, Vice President of Operations
Frigidaire Company

Mark Thompson, President
Kroger

Jack Vaughn, Chairman
Opryland Lodging Group

C. D. Wells, President and CEO
Aerostructure Corporation

Ray Zimmerman, Chairman
Service Merchandise Co., Inc.

BAPTIST HOSPITAL FOUNDATION OF NASHVILLE, INC. BOARD MEMBERS

Scott Jenkins
Rev. James W. Owen Jr.
C. David Stringfield
Arthur D. Victorine
Andrew Benedict
Joe Casey Jr.
Cal MacKay
Dennis Harrison

BAPTIST HOSPITAL FOUNDATION MAJOR DONORS

Abbott Laboratories
Abbott Laboratories Fund
ABG Caulking Contractors, Inc.
Acuff & Associates, Inc.
Affiliated Creditors, Inc.
American Constructors, Inc.
American Healthcorp, Inc.
American Paper & Twine Co.
Anatomic & Clinical Laboratories Associates, P.C.
Anesthesia Medical Group, P.C.
Anonymous Donor
AT&T
Baird Co.
Baker, Donelson, Bearman, Caldwell
Baptist DeKalb Hospital
Baptist Hospital Medical Staff
Baptist Hospital Volunteers
Bates, Guy
Bennett, George
Bluegrass Art Cast, Inc.
Burrus, George Robert
Burrus, Swan B., M.D.
Carter, Oscar W., M.D.
Carter-Spalding-Nesbitt
Charlotte Women's Professional Basketball
Concrete Form Erectors
Danner Foundation
DePuy
Ed's Supply
Estate of Goebel G. Bunch
Ethicon Endo-Surgery

Evans Hailey Mechanical
Fassler, Cheryl Ann, M.D.
Finch, William Tyree, M.D.
First American National Bank
Fowler, Adelaide
Fowler, Ben, III
Freedom Forum World Center
Frost-Arnett Company
General Electric Medical Systems
Goldman, Sachs and Company
Hamilton, Addie
Hannah, Gene A., M.D.
Hardaway Construction Corp. of Tennessee
Hardaway, L. Hall, Jr.
Harris, Charles R.
Hartness, William Owen, M.D.
Hasty, Norman D., M.D.
Hays, James W., M.D.
Hemmer, Gerald
Hernik, Martha M.
Hutton, Robert M., M.D.
IVAC Corporation
King & Ballow
Koch, Debby Patterson
Laserscope Surgical Systems
J. T. Lovell Company
Lovvorn, H. Newton, M.D.
Magnetek, Inc.
Mal-Gar Service Co. Inc.
Mandrell, Irby and Mary
Mariner Health Care, Inc.

Marion Merrell Dow, Inc.
R. C. Mathews Contractor, Inc.
Maxwell, G. Patrick, M.D.
Mayes, Charles E., M.D.
McDermott, Will & Emery
Merck and Company, Inc.
Metro Medical Supply, Inc.
Metropolitan Life
Miles, Louise Mott
Miller Medical Group
Moore, Paul W.
Morehead, V. Tupper, M.D.
Morrison's Hospitality Group
MRC Group
Nashville Banner
Nashville Bridge Co.
Nashville Gastrointestinal Specialists, Inc.
Nashville Machine Company
Nashville Oncology-Hematology Consultants
Nashville Otolaryngology, P.A.
NationsBank
Neurosurgical Group of Nashville
Odom, Harrell, II, M.D.
Oldham, Richard R., M.D.
Olsen, Martha
Otis Elevator
Otology Group
Overfield, Ronald E., M.D.
Owen, Gladys Stringfield
Owens & Minor, Inc.
Pennington, Thomas G., M.D.
Pfizer, Inc.
Phynque, Inc.
Powell Building Group
Powell, James J.
Powell, Sandra G.

Powers, Vern
Purity Dairy Products
Radiology Associates of Nashville
Ross, Kenneth L.
Rowland, Martha L.
Rudy, Jeanette C.
William L. Samples Company
Sedgwick James of Missouri, Inc.
Skojac, Debbie
Smith & Nephew Dyonics, Inc.
Smith Seckman Reid, Inc.
Specialty Surgical Instrumentation, Inc.
Staubach Company
Sterile Design
Stringfield, C. David
Surgical Group of Nashville, P.C.
Tennessee Orthopedic Associates, P.A.
Thomas Nelson, Inc.
Thym, Mary Davenport
Trabue, Sturdivant & DeWitt
Travis, Elizabeth and Randy
Tudor, John M., M.D.
Turner, Jack B.
Urology Associates
Valleylab, Inc.
Louise Bullard Wallace Foundation
WASCO, Inc.
Willis Corroon
Winters, James H.
Winwood, Steve
Wolfe & Travis
Wolfe-Travis Electric
Women's Health Group of Nashville, P.C.
Wray, Taylor M., M.D.
Xerox Co.

INDEX

Page numbers in bold type indicate photo captions.

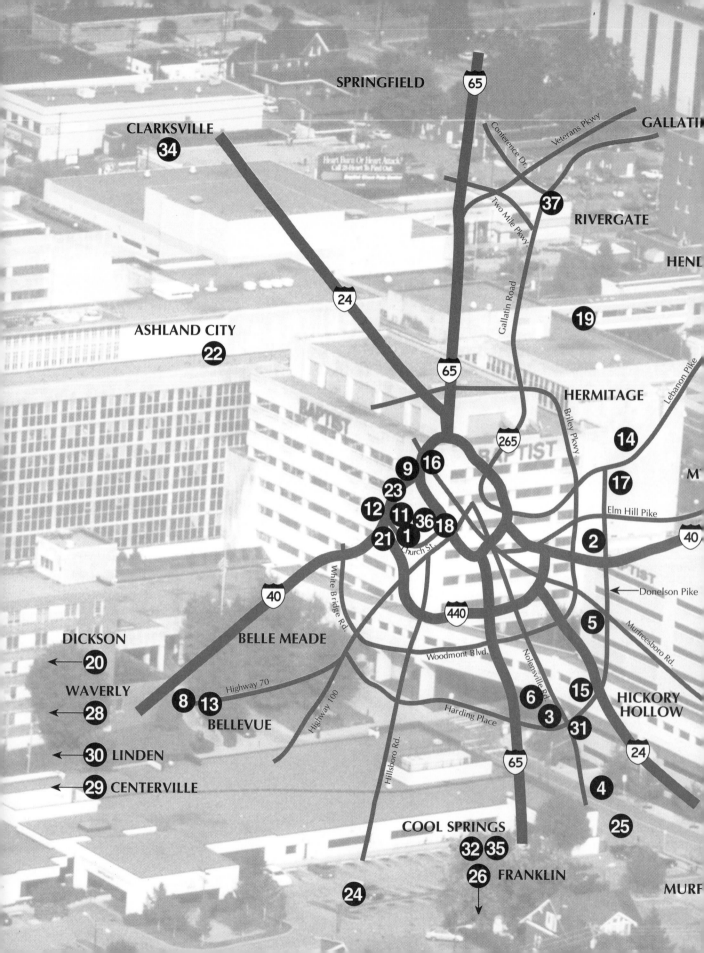